MORE PRAISE FOR
THE BATTLE FOR VETERANS' HEALTHCARE

"Suzanne Gordon has been able to look past the sensational headlines about the VA to the true challenges and opportunities for our nation's veterans. In doing so she reveals the enormous good the VA has done—the innovation, the lives saved, and the promises kept—while acknowledging the tough work ahead to ensure that it fully lives up to its mission."
—Congressman Beto O'Rourke

"Women Veterans have been left out of the debate about the future of the VA health care system. Suzanne Gordon does not make that mistake. As a woman veteran I urge you to read this important book."
—Diane Reppun
Bronze Star-OEF, Founding member Fighting for Veterans Health Care, Lifetime Member of Disabled American Veterans

"Suzanne Gordon has rare clarity and insight into the multiple health risks and problems that veterans face as a result of their military service. She understands that "veterans healthcare" is very different from caring for civilians in the private sector. The Veterans Health Administration has sensitivity to military culture, and special expertise training relevant to the problems veterans experience throughout their lives. Buy this book and read it carefully so you can increase awareness of what must be done for those men and women who have placed life and limb on the line in defense of the Constitution."
—Rick Weidman
Executive Director for Policy & Government Affairs , Vietnam Veterans of America (VVA)

"As a combat veteran who has worked as a psychologist in the VA system for over 28 years, I have experienced the extraordinary changes the VHA has undertaken to provide Veterans with some of the best healthcare available in the US. I have also seen how the VA's dedicated caregivers have been attacked and their critical work denigrated in the press and on Capitol Hill. That's why Suzanne Gordon's compelling account of how the Veterans Health Administration really works could not be more timely. This important compilation of facts, critical analyses, and powerful arguments will give readers a firm foundation for reconsidering the true value of the VHA to our nation. Her book provides a map for taking action to save and improve this invaluable resource."
—**Edgardo Padin-Rivera**
served as Chief of Psychology and Coordinator of Mental Health Services, Louis Stokes Cleveland VA Medical Center

THE BATTLE FOR VETERANS' HEALTHCARE

THE BATTLE FOR VETERANS' HEALTHCARE

Dispatches from the Frontlines of Policy Making and Patient Care

SUZANNE GORDON

CORNELL PUBLISHING
Ithaca

First published 2017 by Cornell Publishing

Printed in the United States of America

A catalog record for this book is available from the Library of Congress
ISBN 978-1-5017-1455-9

FOR

RUSSELL, REBECCA, LOU, AND JUDI

TABLE OF CONTENTS

FOREWORD

IN THE YEARS FOLLOWING THE WAR IN VIETNAM, the Department of Veterans Affairs (VA) healthcare system was viewed by many as a bleak backwater of inefficiency, indifference, and incompetence. Critics cast the VA as a symbol of ineffective and bloated government bureaucracy, and it became the poster child for those who argued that government can never do anything right. However—and remarkably to many—the VA's image began to dramatically change in the late 1990s and continuing into the early 2000s. Among other notable publications, the *Wall Street Journal*, *BusinessWeek*, *New York Times*, *Forbes*, and *Time* began applauding the VA for improvements in the quality of its healthcare services, its pioneering use of information technology, and a newfound responsiveness to veterans. Increasingly, the Veterans Healthcare System was touted as a model for twenty-first-century healthcare—a model, it was argued, that private-sector hospitals and health plans should emulate. Unfortunately, missteps by the VA in recent years have led some politicians and members of the media to suggest that the VA has returned to its post-Vietnam era state of functioning—and that they were right all along about government programs. In this book, Suzanne Gordon highlights why these views miss the mark.

In spite of some now well-described problems, the VA operates one of the nation's best healthcare systems. Studies in leading professional journals continue to document that the quality of VA healthcare is equal and often superior to the care provided in the private sector and that most VA users are very satisfied with their care. Of course, just as in the private sector, there are variations in the quality of services provided by individual VA hospitals and across caregivers, and these variations should be addressed.

In addition to providing good healthcare, the VA Healthcare System conducts cutting-edge research, trains more healthcare professionals than any other institution in America, and plays a critical role in responding to the nation's public health emergencies. In these and other ways that its critics typically overlook, the VA materially benefits all Americans.

As undersecretary for health in the Department of Veterans Affairs and chief executive officer of the Veterans Healthcare System from 1994 to 1999, I had the privilege of leading a team of highly dedicated professionals in a far-reaching initiative to re-engineer VA healthcare. We sought to transform the Veterans Healthcare System into a high-performing organization. We did this by implementing a focused and meaningful performance management system, decentralizing day-to-day operational decision making, moving to a value-based resource allocation system, nurturing innovation, and modernizing information management, including deploying the most effective electronic health record in the world at the time.

We pushed for legislative changes, which allowed the VA to treat all the health problems a veteran might be experiencing—not just those that were service connected—so that we could put the veteran at the center of the healthcare universe and design robust veteran-centered services rooted on a foundation of primary care. We understood that medical and mental health problems not related to military service inevitability impact a veteran's service-connected problems as well as all other aspects of his or her life. We also established important partnerships with private-sector healthcare organizations, partnering with and learning from them, as they did from us. We moved the system from one that provided mostly inpatient hospital care to one that focused increasingly on providing coordinated, community-based ambulatory care. Perhaps most important, we did all we could to support the dedicated VA staff at the frontlines of care.

Since the late 1990s, the VA has been widely recognized as being a pioneer in integrating and coordinating services for veterans, a large number of whom have highly complex medical and psychological conditions caused or exacerbated by military service. Primary care—which has been integrated with mental health care, as well as with pharmacy, nutrition, social work, housing, and employment services—has become the foundation of the VA healthcare system. While still a work in progress, the VA has sought to weave a healing web of interconnected programs and support services because it recognizes that the complex conditions that affect many veterans must be treated in a holistic, whole-person manner, rather than as a collage of disparate clinical conditions. This way of viewing healthcare service delivery is only now beginning to be operationalized in the private sector.

The VA has also become a leading advocate for and innovator in patient safety, patient engagement, and team-based care. VA physicians, nurses, and allied healthcare professionals work together in collaborative and complementary ways to meet the needs of their patients, and they continually seek new and better ways to do so. The VA has funded and supported system-wide deployment of innovative approaches to veteran-centric care—innovations often conceptualized and developed on the frontlines of care delivery. The VA has sought to develop a multilane innovation highway that is facilitated by it being a national system of care—in fact, America's only national healthcare system.

Regrettably, during the past decade or so, the culture of quality improvement and accountability that had taken root in VA healthcare in the late 1990s began to crack and erode. A gradual return to highly centralized control of operational decision making, misguided approaches to performance measurement, growing insularity, and burgeoning bureaucracy all chipped away and undermined the culture of quality that had taken hold in the late 1990s. Too often, VA leaders have lost sight of the sacred mission underlying the Veterans Healthcare System. And while the quality of clinical care generally has remained high, these regressive trends negatively impacted the provision of services in some instances.

VA's organizational retrenchments have prompted some to again call for veterans' healthcare to be turned over to the private sector. Fortunately, more knowledgeable and dispassionate persons have spoken out against this idea, understanding that privatizing veterans' healthcare would be a grave mistake and would not serve our former warriors well.

Instead of privatizing veterans' healthcare, we should focus on fixing VA's problems, many of which also plague private-sector healthcare providers. Indeed, stories reported in newspapers and other media remind us every day of the shortcomings of private-sector healthcare, and especially when it comes to treating mental health problems, coordinating care for complex medical conditions, and treating socioeconomically disadvantaged persons. Clearly, privatizing veterans' healthcare offers no panacea.

In this book Suzanne Gordon wisely counsels us that we must view the VA's problems in their historical and cultural context. She reminds us that modern healthcare is extremely complex and that a wide-angle lens should be used to get a complete picture of a healthcare system. For example, consider the issue of wait times in the VA. Without question, the VA has had serious problems with wait times at many of its medical centers in recent years, and unfortunately, it did not appropriately manage these problems. However, wait times are a significant problem in the private sector as well. And when considering wait times, one also should reflect on the quality of care that is being waited for. In this regard I am reminded of the findings of a recent study that some colleagues and I undertook to assess variations in the quality of care for cancer among Californians with different types of health insurance. We found that veterans waited longer for their treatment than patients with other forms of health insurance, but they also had generally better outcomes than comparable patients having other types of health insurance, and their treatment was more likely to be appropriate for their condition. This should not be taken to mean that the VA should ignore its wait time problems. Clearly, the VA needs to see many of its patients more quickly, but the fact that the VA's cancer care outcomes were better, notwithstanding the delays in patients getting care, underscores the importance of getting the right care. As important as wait times are, they should not be the only metric by which a health system is measured.

This book also points out that when VA healthcare is reported upon, it is often held to performance standards not equally applied to private providers. For example, when the VA suffers from a shortage of primary-care physicians or psychiatrists, it is castigated for failing to fill staff vacancies without regard to the fact that a national shortage of these professionals has created similar problems for many other health systems, and that the government's below-market-value salaries materially confound the VA's efforts to attract limited-supply medical specialists. Or, when a veteran becomes addicted to opioid pain killers or comes into the VA after having become addicted while on active duty, the VA caregivers are blamed for overusing these drugs without regard to the current national epidemic of opioid overuse and the fact that healthcare providers everywhere are struggling to find ways to adequately manage pain without using too many opioid drugs. Similarly, when the VA spends a pittance on artwork or an aquarium to help create a comforting and soothing environment in its facilities, it is attacked for wasting money, while private-sector hospitals are lauded and celebrated for spending much greater amounts to decorate their lobbies and hallways. Clearly, the VA's shortcomings cannot be overlooked or excused because similar problems exist in other healthcare settings, but a more balanced and constructive conversation would be less demoralizing to the thousands of VA employees who go above and beyond the call of duty to provide veterans with high-quality care.

The backbone of the VA Healthcare System is its army of highly dedicated clinicians, administrators, and other healthcare workers—over a third of which are veterans themselves. These dedicated professionals are committed to providing high-quality care to veterans, often forgoing much more lucrative careers in the private sector out of a desire to serve fellow veterans. Instead of denigrating and disparaging these committed professionals, our elected leaders should help them succeed in a system that is too often challenged by unnecessarily complicated government rules and cumbersome processes, inadequate funding, and unrealistic expectations. I know from my tenure with the VA that, if appropriately supported and led, the VA's dedicated staff will provide a level of service and care that millions of Americans can only wish they would receive from their healthcare providers.

The Honorable Kenneth W. Kizer, MD, MPH
Distinguished Professor, University of California Davis School of Medicine and Betty Irene Moore School of Nursing
Director, Institute for Population Health Improvement, UC Davis Health
Sacramento, California

PREFACE

OVER THE LAST THREE YEARS, a campaign to dismantle and ulti-mately privatize the Veterans Health Administration (VHA) has gained momentum. Funded by far-right Libertarians like the Koch brothers, this effort has caught on in Congress and has even been supported by some Democrats. It has also been aided and abetted by unfair reporting and editorializing in some of our nation's leading media. With the election of Donald J. Trump, the threats facing the VHA are part of a larger attack on publicly funded healthcare in America.

As a journalist covering healthcare issues for the last thirty years, in June of 2014 I embarked on research for a larger book about innovations in the delivery of care at the VHA and spent nearly three years observing VHA caregivers and programs and talking to veterans and their families. Having seen the high-quality care that the VHA delivers and the commu-nity of care it has established for both patients and caregivers, I was struck not only by the speed at which the anti-VHA campaign has accelerated but also by the false and misleading claims made to discredit its work. Above all, I've been alarmed by the serious consequences that VHA privatization would have, not just for the more than nine million veterans—and their families—who depend on its services. Innovations in care at the VHA, as well as its research and teaching of the almost 300,000 people who work in the system, benefit us all. In fact, the integrated care the VHA delivers to veterans should be a model for improving our larger American health-care system, which suffers from fragmentation and lack of coordination, unnecessary treatment, and other problems and inefficiencies.

The VHA, of course, has its own problems: lack of access and overly long wait times in some facilities, as well as poor administration. Much of the debate about the future of the VHA fails to situate these problems in their historical context or to understand how they reflect larger societal priorities. Difficulty recruiting staff at the VHA is a result of the chronic congressional underfunding of the nation's largest healthcare system. It is also a result of decisions made by the larger healthcare system to focus on the overproduction of medical specialists rather than an appropriate balance between primary-care and generalist physicians and specialists. Problems with mismanagement are not unique to government bureaucra-cies. The private sector, where companies like General Motors, Volkswagen, Wells Fargo, and the Cleveland Clinic are only a few recent examples in a long list of corporate malfeasance and lack of transparency and accountability, is rife with these problems.

Delays in getting services to veterans in need also have to do with cumbersome and difficult-to-understand eligibility requirements that Congress has imposed to limit the number of veterans who are eligible for VHA healthcare or other VA benefits. As former VHA Undersecretary for Health Kenneth W. Kizer has written, many of these problems can and must be solved, but their solution is not privatization of the VHA.[1]

Over the last few years, as I have read poorly reported stories about the VHA and analyzed a slew of misguided proposals for reforming the system, I have written a series of commentaries for newspapers, magazines, and blogs based on my own research and interviews with veterans and their caregivers. I am still working on a longer book about the innovative clinical care and treatment models that the VHA has developed, but in the meantime, I have pulled together an edited collection of my VHA-related pieces. It's my hope that this primer will add information and analysis often missing from the current debate over the VHA and its future.[1]

My VHA coverage has been inspired by getting to know veterans like the one who wrote a letter to the VA Commission on Care, whose work is discussed in Section Two. In April 2016 I posted this eloquent letter on my blog and then received an email from the veteran's wife, which I include in Appendix A. His letter, which I excerpt here, illustrates what is at stake in the fight about veterans' healthcare and why I feel compelled to speak up for veterans who depend on VHA services as well as the many devoted caregivers who assist them.

From: [redacted]
To: Commission on Care
Subject: [EXTERNAL] Iraq War Veteran Date: Sunday, April 17, 2016 1:57:49 AM

---

1 Because these dispatches were written as events developed, I have combined some to avoid repetition. I indicate at the end of the book where the articles originally appeared. I ask for the reader's forbearance for the inevitable redundancies that may creep in. I also use the term "VHA" throughout this short book when I mean just that—the Veterans Health Administration. I do this because so many people confuse the VHA with the Veterans Benefit Administration, too often attributing the problems created by the latter with experiences they have had with the former.

Dear Commission on Care Members

I'm writing this in hopes to make you understand that the VA is more than a place that Veterans just get their health care at. Also I hope that my story will make you understand that the VA is more than worth saving because the VA saved ME! . . .

My VA story begins with me coming home from Iraq in 2007 . . . I knew something was wrong but I didn't know what . . . felt like a stranger to myself. I couldn't sleep at night. I was hearing gun fire in my sleep, waking up looking for my rifle, getting up and putting on my uniform during thunder storms. I was angry all the time with inappropriate outbursts, having crying spells. My brain was always going and I couldn't figure out how to shake this out of my head . . . I started to drink to try to cope with this person I have become . . .

One day I received a call from an amazing social worker informing me that I was assigned to him and that he wanted to set up an appointment to get me started in my VA care. So I set up the appointment . . . On the day of the appointment I was marked as a no show because I was drunk and in my basement. The next day I received another phone call from the social worker informing me that I missed my appointment . . . that I needed to come in. So we set up another appointment and I did the same thing and no showed again . . . Finally I had enough and said okay I will come in if you stop calling me. So I made the appointment but this time I showed up because that weekend I found myself drunk in my basement with a rope around my neck ready to kill myself . . . And that was the start of the VA Health Care Saving my life. Not just mine but many Veterans like me that I met on my journey at the VA of figuring out who I was and what happened to the person I used to be . . .

I want to ask this committee since we know what's wrong with the VA do you know what is right? What is right is that my experience is something that comes with much sacrifice and the VA is the only place I feel safe with it. I am surrounded by men and women that know what serving our country really means...that really understand the cost to keep this country safe.

So to your solution of sending us to private healthcare providers is the wrong direction because the VA is filled with veteran and staff that have raised their right hands and said!

"I, do solemnly swear that I will support and defend the Constitution of the United States against all enemies, foreign and domestic; that I will bear true faith and allegiance to the same; and that I will obey the orders of the President of the United States and the orders of the officers appointed over me, according to regulations and the Uniform Code of Military Justice. So help me God."

There is no private health care provider office that can offer me this type of care. So just fix our VA because it belongs to us not to the private sector.

Thank You Iraq Veteran

The stakes in this battle for veterans' healthcare involve more than veterans. Those affected include veterans' family members as well as those who work at the VHA, many of whom are veterans themselves. But finally, what is at issue is the future of healthcare—not just medical treatment—in the United States. If we refuse to care for veterans and view them only as another profit center, how can we possibly learn to care for each other when we are sick and vulnerable?

SECTION ONE

THE VA AND ITS CRITICS

ALTHOUGH THERE HAS BEEN A TORRENT of news and debate about the Veterans Health Administration since July 2014, when wait-time problems at the Phoenix VA Health Care System and some other facilities became big news, very few members of the public (and, it appears, even fewer member of the media or Congress) understand what the VHA is and does, how it differs from, say, the Veterans Benefit Administration, how many veterans it actually serves, what its mission includes, and how its services compare with the private-sector healthcare providers with which it is increasingly asked to compete.

As we shall see, media coverage—as well as the debate on Capitol Hill—has focused almost exclusively on the negative. The media has neglected critical questions like how private-sector providers stack up when it comes to wait times or providing appropriate medical and mental health services (not just to veterans but civilian patients). One of the most important questions that is almost never addressed is whether private-sector providers are ready to serve the nation's veterans when they are doing such a poor job serving nonveteran patients. This section of the book explores what the VHA does, how it performs, and why it has come under such heavy attack over the last several years.

CHAPTER ONE
HOW THE VHA WORKS

ON A BEAUTIFUL, SUNNY DAY IN 2015, as part of my current research on patient care at the Veterans Health Administration (VHA), I tagged along with an occupational therapist named Heather Freitag. She works for the VHA's Home-Based Primary Care program (HBPC) at the San Francisco VA Health Care System (SFVAHCS) and was making her first visit to a 79-year-old Korean War veteran suffering from dementia.

The man's wife, only five years younger, was clearly overwhelmed by the burden of caring for him by herself while dealing with her own mounting health problems. For more than an hour, Freitag scrutinized every niche and cranny of their tidy bungalow in the Excelsior District.

The VHA caregiver quickly discovered that her patient's narrow, sagging bed made it too difficult for his wife to turn him. In his frail condition, the two-inch lip around their shower stall had also become an insurmountable obstacle to daily bathing. The veteran's lack of mobility had already resulted in two small bedsores that could—if not properly treated—lead to serious infection and costly hospitalization.

The goal of Freitag's primary-care team is to prevent such problems. They try to keep patients comfortable and where most would like to remain—in their own home for as long as possible. After returning to her office, Freitag put in an order for a special bariatric hospital bed, complete with a state-of-the-art air mattress. She also began designing a plastic chair that would ease the man's difficulty with home shower access.

In caring for this veteran, the HBPC would dispatch to the same San Francisco address a physician, a nurse-practitioner, a nutritionist, a geriatric psychologist, and a physical therapist. And, of course, they would be supplemented by home healthcare aides (the only providers I could ever expect to see under similar circumstances when utilizing my own, privately funded, long term–care insurance sometime in the future). Indeed, for most elderly shut-ins, home-care workers are the main caregivers who render heroic critical services that help people function in daily life.

Such carefully coordinated, high-quality care may be unusual elsewhere, but it is not a rarity at the VHA. In the years I've spent visiting VHA hospitals and clinics all over the country, I've found it to be the norm. While observing primary-care providers and geriatricians, palliative care and hospice specialists, mental health practitioners, designers of prosthetic devices, medical and nursing researchers, and experts in team training and patient safety, I've also interviewed veterans of all ages and their family members. Every healthcare system has its critics and complainers, but in thirty years of writing about the interaction between patients and providers, I've never seen better institutional support for those who deliver patient care.

Sadly, since 2014, the sustained attack by conservative ideologues has turned the public against the VHA, a healthcare system that most members of the public, media, and policy community don't understand. In fact, confusion about veterans' healthcare is so common that many veterans themselves don't understand which branch of the Department of Veterans Affairs, or of the government, is responsible for either their good or bad experiences or their ability to access services and benefits. Many think that the Department of Veterans Affairs, commonly known as the VA, is actually one unified agency, when in fact it is comprised of three different branches. There's the VHA, which is the healthcare system. Then there's the Veterans Benefits Administration (VBA), which determines who is eligible for what benefits, including the Medical Benefits Package, disability compensation, pensions, the GI Bill, survivor benefits, and home loans, among other things. Then there's the National Cemetery Administration, which is in charge of burials and cemeteries. Another central player in VHA healthcare is the Department of Defense (DOD), which issues discharges from the military and determines the various discharge categories that underpin eligibility for VHA healthcare. In many instances veterans attribute delays in getting healthcare to the VHA when the holdup may be with the VBA or the Defense Department's determination of a veteran's discharge status.

A RESEARCH AND TEACHING POWERHOUSE

With its salaried staff of about 250,000 (a third of whom are veterans themselves), the VHA is the nation's largest (and only publicly funded), fully integrated healthcare system. Its 150 hospitals, 819 clinics, 300 mental health centers, and other facilities—many located in rural areas that the private sector ignores—care for more than 230,000 people a day. As Phillip Longman described in his book, *The Best Care Anywhere: Why VA Health Care Would Work Better for Everyone,* the VHA was the first healthcare system to develop, implement, and embrace the kind of healthcare information technology that other hospitals and health systems are now trying—with far less success—to utilize.[2]

The VHA has three primary missions: patient care, teaching, and research. Since 1946 the VHA has affiliated with major academic teaching hospitals and now trains over 70 percent of American physicians as well as students and trainees in forty other healthcare professions. The VHA's large number of enrollees has enabled it to become a research powerhouse that produces scientific advances benefiting all Americans, not just veterans. To cite just two examples, the VHA, in partnership with the National

Institutes of Health, conducted the studies to prove that the shingles vaccine—which millions of senior citizens now take—was indeed safe for all Americans. VHA researchers also did pioneering work documenting a reduction in post-surgical mortality when patients with known cardiac risks were given beta blockers before surgery. Now this is standard practice not only for veterans, but for all patients who undergo surgery. The VHA performed the first successful liver transplant and developed the nicotine patch. It recently launched the Million Veteran Program to study how genes impact health. Needless to say, findings will not be limited to the use of veterans alone.

PATIENTS WHO ARE OLDER AND SICKER

With the exception of Medicare or Medicaid (which are not integrated delivery systems), no other healthcare system cares for as many old and poor patients as the VHA. Because of the timing of America's participation in various wars, when you go into a waiting room at a VHA hospital or clinic anywhere in the country, you will not see a mix of older and younger patients. In many VHA facilities, you'll see a bunch of guys proudly wearing baseball caps that say "Vietnam Veteran," or "Korean War Veteran." There will even be the occasional octogenarian or even nonagenarian, but very few people under forty.

In 2012 the average veteran patient was sixty-two. Older people, of course, are more challenging to treat, and vets have more medical conditions than nonveterans in the same age cohort. And the VHA has provided more geriatric services to these veterans than are available in the private sector in spite of the fact that America is dealing with a larger proportion of aging patients.

In 1991 one report on VHA care stated that the VA has pioneered what is for Americans a unique continuum of treatment programs to meet the needs of the elderly and other veteran patients who require long-term care. In addition to traditional acute and ambulatory care services, it provides a broad range of institutional and noninstitutional long-term programs for patients who are not able to live independently. These services include palliative and hospice care; nursing home and adult day health care; hospital-based home care; domiciliary and community residential care; and respite care.[3]

The VHA has since pioneered fellowships in geriatric care and produced programs and research in critical conditions and treatments impacting older patients. Long before the cost-effectiveness of palliative and hospice care was recognized elsewhere, the VHA was providing some of the best services in the country to people with advanced and terminal illnesses.

The VHA also has one of the most extensive systems of mental health care in a country where the treatment of the mentally ill is a national scandal. Many combat veterans may have physical and mental illnesses for which they need treatment—in fact, veterans suffer from mental illness at a higher rate than the general population and also have a higher rate of chronic illness. An estimated 16 to 30 percent of combat veterans, for example, have post-traumatic stress disorder (PTSD), as do many female veterans who have been victims of military sexual trauma. Although it took the federal government far too long to officially recognize PTSD, VHA psychologists, psychiatrists, and social workers have helped develop pioneering treatments—cognitive behavioral therapy and prolonged exposure therapy—that are the gold standard for anyone suffering from PTSD today.

The VHA is now dealing with the epidemic of opiate abuse that now plagues the country by pioneering programs in integrated pain management. These programs use various methods—including mindfulness meditation, yoga, massage, and classes in pain management—to wean veterans from narcotics. Through its Veterans Integration into Academic Leadership (VITAL) program, as well as many others, the VHA is also trying to help veterans navigate the tricky passage as they leave the military and try to readjust to civilian life.[4] Although this is a serious problem for veterans who have been in combat, it is also one for veterans who may never have left the continental United States. The VHA has also launched many suicide-prevention initiatives, including the Veterans Crisis Line. Suicide-prevention coordinators at every VHA medical center train every employee—no matter what level in the healthcare hierarchy—how to recognize signs that suggest that a veteran is at risk for suicide. The VHA also has programs that identify such veterans and target them for special outreach and attention.

Apart from Medicaid, no other healthcare system in the United States treats as many low-income patients—many of whom are unemployed and homeless, not to mention mentally and physically ill or abusing drugs, alcohol, and other substances. The Department of Veterans Affairs provides not only healthcare services to these low-income or homeless veterans but also social and legal support. In 2012 the department launched its Housing First program to assure that even veterans who were abusing alcohol or drugs or had other unaddressed healthcare needs could find shelter, which will hopefully make it possible for them to address other serious health problems. The VA has also helped to pioneer a system of Veterans Courts, which help veterans with legal problems avoid or limit incarceration.

The VHA is also the pace setter in diagnosing and developing new understanding of traumatic brain injury (TBI) and chronic traumatic encephalopathy; its institutional research and knowledge are now benefiting victims of pro football concussions occurring far from any foreign battlefields. Its Polytrauma System of Care is also pioneering new methods of rehabilitation for TBI. The VHA is a leader in the use of telemedicine for patients suffering from both mental and physical illness—a development recently featured in *The New York Times* (without, of course, mentioning the VHA's leadership in the field).

The VHA has also recognized the needs of increasing numbers of female veterans (80 percent of whom have experienced some form of military sexual trauma) and has created a system of women's health clinics, which have their own separate spaces within larger facilities.

The VHA is sometimes accused of failing to reach out to and welcome new veterans as patients. The real culprit is, however, Congress, which keeps failing to provide the VHA with adequate funding and is constantly narrowing and tightening eligibility requirements. Although some outreach efforts may have lagged in some specific places, I have been repeatedly impressed by the amount of work that is done on a daily basis to recruit new patients and make sure those already enrolled have full access to services. For example, I followed a VHA social worker who spends her days patrolling the streets of San Francisco trying to find homeless veterans not yet connected to the VA. She and other social workers all over the country also make sure that veterans in board-and-care homes, shelters, and transitional housing facilities are not being exploited by unscrupulous "entrepreneurs" who prey on the poor, mentally ill, and homeless.

In West Haven, Connecticut, I visited a remarkable program called the Errera Community Care Center. The Errera Center provides intensive services for mentally ill and homeless veterans, finding them permanent shelter and also helping them find jobs and connecting them to primary-care medical providers. Over and over again, in VHA hospitals and clinics all over the country, I have watched clerks, nurses, and primary-care providers practically walk veterans to appointments, call them to remind them about services that are available to them, and even visit their homes to make sure they are safe.

At the West Haven VA, I spent a day at one of the system's thirteen Blind Rehabilitation Centers. These residential facilities serve some of the 157,000 veterans who are legally blind and the one million whose vision is so impaired that they have difficulty navigating daily life. There, I met veterans whose private-sector ophthalmologists or optometrists often sent them away, saying, "There is nothing further to be done," spend weeks in an inpatient residential program learning how to function in daily life. In the VHA system, therapists have themselves spent hours wearing goggles or glasses that simulate the vision problems of their patients. They thus become better prepared to teach their patients how to walk with a cane, cook, do leather- or woodwork, or use computer programs that are specially designed for the vision-impaired. When patients are ready to return home, they take special microwaves, iPads, iPhones, computers, or other equipment with them, courtesy of the VHA. The private sector does not offer any similar inpatient residential program with such extensive benefits.

THE WARS IN IRAQ AND AFGHANISTAN

Veterans from the recent wars in Iraq and Afghanistan suffer from battle-related trauma that may, in the years to come, dwarf the physical and mental health problems of those who served in Vietnam. Because of the military's successful system of battlefield hospitals and triage, these young men and women have survived trauma and injury that would have been fatal in prior conflicts. And because of their combat experiences and multiple tours of duty, many also suffer from PTSD, TBI, and perhaps even amputations—in other words, polytrauma. One in six veterans who served in these conflicts also has a substance-abuse problem.

The VHA has waived its standard eligibility requirements and is providing care to post–9/11 veterans for five years after they leave the military. After that it will continue to provide care for any service-related conditions.

Some of the veterans I have interviewed include men who have lost a leg or an arm and been fitted with state-of-the-art prosthetics for both daily and athletic use. Others—like a 28-year-old who spends his nights at home on guard duty, patrolling the perimeter of his property by checking the locks on the doors to make sure no one can get in—may receive intensive, inpatient treatment for PTSD. None of this would be available in the private sector.

In 2010 the VHA launched a program to support home-based caregivers who are tending to post–9/11 veterans with mental or chronic physical illnesses. In our larger healthcare system, family caregivers are essentially on their own when they care for a loved one who has a major mental health or physical disability. Many are rewarded for their service by loss of jobs or promotions and may eventually sacrifice their own health because of the emotional and physical stress of their caregiving burden. The program provides these caregivers with training, supportive services—including mental health counseling—and even financial stipends to help them shoulder their burdens. Why does the VHA take on this long-term commitment? Because it has a lifelong commitment to its patients and their families, it recognizes that it is cost-effective to help keep the veteran in his or her home rather than paying for hospital or nursing-home care.

ELIGIBILITY LABYRINTH

Most members of the public think that all veterans are eligible for VHA services. Nothing could be further from the truth. Because Congress has not allocated funds sufficient to provide healthcare for all 22 million or more Americans who served in the military, the VHA must enforce eligibility rules that restrict care to the sickest and poorest veterans while excluding more affluent and healthy ones. To be among the nine million vets who currently qualify for the VHA's full Medical Benefits Package, applicants must have an honorable discharge. Not all eligible veterans have seen combat, but all of them—if they served after 1980—must provide evidence of a "service-connected disability."

The level of service connection can range from 0 to 100 percent. A partial disability finding might result from back or knee injuries incurred while carrying 60 to 100-pound packs during basic training or combat—a problem few civilians connect to military service. Other, more serious, conditions warranting VHA coverage include amyotrophic lateral sclerosis (or Lou Gehrig's disease) or other diseases that were a side effect of Agent Orange exposure during the Vietnam War and the TBI and amputations suffered by targets of improvised explosive devices in Iraq or Afghanistan. VHA and DOD researchers are also discovering that many service members, like football players who suffer repeated concussions, are suffering from mild TBI because of the exposure to blast pressure from firing heavy weaponry.[6]

One large group of veterans excluded from VHA services and the broader array of VA benefits is the 125,000 or more who received an "other than honorable" discharge from the armed forces. Many of these vets suffer from mental or physical illnesses arising from their military service; their allegedly dishonorable behavior while on active duty may even have been triggered by a job-related health condition. Some were simply mustered out unfairly—during the era of Don't Ask, Don't Tell or before it—because of their sexual orientation. Yet all are ineligible for any VA benefits from the GI bill to healthcare to homeless services and more because of the discharge characterization the Department of Defense assigned them when they separated from military service, which the VA has accepted.

In civilian life, a worker who gets fired, with or without just cause, doesn't automatically lose current or future access to state workers' compensation systems. Eligibility for partial compensation for lost income caused by job-related injuries or illnesses and related medical insurance coverage for those conditions is not contingent on someone having a good work record, although employers can contest claims on the grounds that they are not job-related. For example, a coal miner applying for state or federal black-lung benefits just has to prove that he or she worked in the industry and supply sufficient medical documentation of resulting lung damage. Disabled miners with a proven diagnosis of pneumoconiosis can't be denied benefits because they were fired from their last job (or fired in other circumstances before that).

This is not how it works in the military, where your discharge characterization determines all. These assigned categories range from "honorable" to the punitive "dishonorable," which can encompass severe crimes as well as bad conduct that is serious but not enough to require a court martial. In the middle spectrum are "other than honorable" discharges—administrative, nonpunitive sanctioning of people with performance or disciplinary problems also not considered serious enough to warrant a court-martial.

The accused, in these cases, may have been drunk on duty, tested positive for drug use, or engaged in fights.

Veterans advocacy groups and attorneys who work on veterans' benefits have identified significant problems with this classification system, which, in the case of "dis-honorable" and "other than honorable" discharges, leads to denial of VHA benefits. Swords to Plowshares, a San Francisco–based advocacy group, notes that the exact same workplace conduct can result in a different type of discharge in different branches of the service. An airman testing positive for drugs might get sent to rehab, complete the program, and get an honorable discharge. A marine corps commander with a zero-tolerance policy may just boot a marine with the same problem right out of the service.

Commanders often fail to consider the full circumstances of an individual's discipline problem. Did the veteran have service-related PTSD or another mental health problem? Was he or she in combat? Where? For how long? Was the female veteran a victim of military sexual trauma who drank because of the abuse? Did a woman report harassment or rape by a senior officer and get kicked out of the service on trumped-up charges?

Because of their discharge characterization, more than eight thousand veterans a year are denied services that many desperately need. Although they can apply for a discharge upgrade from the DOD, these appeals are rarely granted. The process of establishing initial eligibility at the VA is also too cumbersome.[7] And veteran advocates argue that the VA could challenge discharge characterizations far more effectively and frequently than it does. Although both the DOD and VA are aware of the problem and trying to address it, Congress is ultimately responsible for the complex set of eligibility requirements and discharge characterizations that unfairly limit veteran access to healthcare and other benefits. Congress could begin to remedy this injustice by, at least, directing the VA to deny eligibility only to veterans with punitive discharges. This would automatically expand access to VA benefits to those with "other than honorable" discharges. If Congress chose to give these veterans the care and service they deserve, it would, of course, also have to allocate the additional funding to pay for these services.

COSTS OF CARE

Although it is difficult to compare VHA care to the private sector because so many veterans have so many more severe problems, one study documented that, using 1999 data, the full range of services the VHA provided would have cost 21 percent more in the private sector. Inpatient care in the private sector would have cost 16 percent more, outpatient care 11 percent more, and prescription drugs a whopping 70 percent more. These estimates were based on Medicare Part A payment methods.[8]

The VHA can produce these savings because the government negotiates lower prices with the pharmaceutical industry and physicians and other healthcare providers are salaried and don't have a financial incentive to overtreat. VHA care is also more focused on prevention, early treatment, and patient's ability to function as independently as possible, which saves money over the long term. And of course, there are no for-profit middlemen, as in the private, partly for-profit, insurance-based system, and the VHA does not waste taxpayer dollars on high executive salaries or expensive marketing and advertising. You will never find a director of a VHA hospital who earned more than $4 million in 2014, like the CEO of the Cleveland Clinic, Delos "Toby" Cosgrove,[9] or $15.4 million like the president of Johns Hopkins Hospital, Ronald Peterson.[10] And Congress does not allow the VHA to engage in the kind of expensive branding campaigns that cost the U.S. taxpayer and American patients billions a year.

Some critics of the VHA insist that it is too costly to provide the level of service I have described. In his Senate testimony on his February 2014 budget request, Bernie Sanders eloquently addressed this critique: "When our men and women come home from war, some wounded in body, some wounded in spirit, I don't want to hear people telling me it's too expensive to take care of those wounded veterans. I don't accept that. If you think it's too expensive to take care of veterans, don't send them to war."[11]

CHAPTER TWO
IGNORING THE FACTS: THE ANTI-VET AGENDA

THE VETERANS HEALTH ADMINISTRATION grew out of Abraham Lincoln's Civil War pledge: "To care for him who shall have borne the battle and for his widow, and his orphan."[12] An independent assessment of the VHA's record on care delivery, conducted by the RAND Corporation and mandated by the 2014 Choice Act, documents that the VHA outperforms the private sector on many measures, is equivalent on some, and marginally worse on only a few

"VA wait times," RAND reported, "do not seem to be substantially worse than non-VA waits." VA patients get care that is often higher quality than that in the private sector—with performance variation "lower than that observed in private sector health plans."[13] A study published recently in JAMA reported that men with heart failure, heart attacks, or pneumonia were less likely to die if treated at a VHA hospital rather than a non-VHA hospital.[14] A recent study reported that women veterans have higher rates of screening for cervical and breast cancer when they see a specially designated women's health provider.[15]

What's more, the VHA is a model of a fully integrated healthcare delivery system. Genuine integration affords veterans a level of care unavailable to most Americans, who remain subject to our fragmented private-sector healthcare system. A VHA patient moving from Boston to San Francisco can get uninterrupted care from professionals with access to his or her medical records. When the same patient sees his or her primary-care practitioner to discuss health problems—diabetes, say, or PTSD—he or she can then walk down the hall and talk to a nutritionist about a diet, a pharmacist about how to correctly administer insulin, or a mental health professional. Services like audiology, physical therapy, or dermatology may be provided to the veteran on the same day in the same place, or even via telemedicine in a VHA facility or in the veteran's home. This explains why, in a recent survey of veterans for the American Customer Satisfaction Index, patients rated the system's services as equal to or better than private-sector healthcare facilities.[16]

Because the VHA is a public entity, its facilities actually display greater accountability—and more transparency to patients and their families—than private healthcare systems. When veterans have a VA-related beef—or in-house whistle-blowers have a tale to tell—they are quick to notify their elected representatives. Such complaints regularly trigger individual constituent service queries from members of Congress or, as is the case today, oversight hearings by House and Senate committees. Good luck triggering a similar rapid response to patient or staff complaints in the private sector!

Consider the example of one Vietnam veteran, retired Air Force Colonel David Antoon, who had surgery for prostate cancer at the Cleveland Clinic in January 2008. The operation was performed with the robotic da Vinci Surgical System. Antoon suffered what he argues were preventable surgical errors, which left him both impotent and incontinent. As a result, he was forced to quit his job as a captain with Delta Airlines.

Antoon alleged that his medical harm was caused because doctors in training, without supervision and without his knowledge or consent, performed the operation and that the surgeon who had agreed to perform the surgery was not present at any time during his surgery or hospitalization, a practice known as "ghost surgery." Antoon tried to hold the institution accountable. He wrote two letters to CEO Toby Cosgrove asking him for an investigation of what had happened to him. Cosgrove never replied. He also lodged a complaint with the Centers for Medicare and Medicaid Services (CMS). Antoon alleged that operating room logs and the Cleveland Clinic audit report of his surgery provide no evidence that the staff surgeon who agreed to perform his surgery was present. When it investigated the incident, CMS's survey notes show that his surgeon was performing multiple surgeries beginning within minutes of each other. CMS also cited the entire urology department for having no credentialing of staff or residents in addition to having no privileging requirements for surgeons to use the da Vinci robot. Antoon also filed a lawsuit against the clinic for malpractice.[17]

In response to Antoon's lawsuit, the Cleveland Clinic said it was not guilty of any wrongdoing. More important, its lawyers argued that Antoon should not even be granted his day in court because he had filed his suit too many years after the surgery. Ohio's Eighth District Court of Appeals ruled in Antoon's favor, and his case was remanded to a jury trial. The Cleveland Clinic appealed this decision to the Ohio Supreme Court. Several of the court's elected justices had taken contributions from the Cleveland Clinic and other medical lobbying groups. The clinic lawyer defending this case before the court hosted and co-chaired fundraising events for two of the justices. After a six-year legal battle, the Ohio Supreme Court sided with the Cleveland Clinic. Antoon called the decision "profoundly unfair" to victims of medical malpractice.

"What was the worst thing about this case," Antoon told me, "is the sense of betrayal. There was no way to hold anyone accountable for what happened in our private, profit-driven system where insurance companies are in the middle, and high-paid CEOs are willing to accept and conceal negative patient outcomes."

For treatment of the permanent medical harm he suffered, Antoon now receives all of his medical care at the Dayton VA Medical Center. Antoon says the quality of care he receives in the VA system is far better, far more efficient, far more transparent, and far more compassionate than what he experienced in the private sector. "The VA system is the model needed for this country—a system where patients and providers have the same goal: positive patient outcomes."

In another irony in this case, when he was chairman of the House Veterans' Affairs Committee, Congressman Jeff Miller, as well as other critics of the VHA, argued that hospital or health system leaders whose institutions are involved in significant patient safety problems should not receive bonuses or salary increases. During Antoon's efforts to remedy problems with the Cleveland Clinic, the institution was under investigation by CMS for serious patient safety problems that went unremedied and almost resulted in its suspension from the Medicare program. Yet between 2010 and 2014, CEO Toby Cosgrove's annual compensation increased from over $2.3 million to over $4 million.[18]

Ignoring the VHA's record of care delivery and that of private-sector providers like the Cleveland Clinic, conservatives have exploited the wait-time problems and delays uncovered in 2014 in Phoenix and some other VHA facilities to argue that the entire VHA system is broken and the VHA should no longer provide healthcare services. They want to eliminate the VHA and transfer veterans to the private-sector healthcare system, with the government serving as payer, rather than provider, of care.

Needless to say, this would be a huge boon to private-sector hospitals, which is why many support this plan. It is also favored by large pharmaceutical and medical equipment companies. Big Pharma has long chafed at the fact that the VHA—unlike, say, Medicare or other U.S. health plans—negotiates lower pharmaceutical prices through its drug formularies. Because VHA physicians and other staff are on salary, they have little financial incentive to either over- or undertreat their patients and thus use medical equipment and treatments much more judiciously than their counterparts in the private sector.

The VHA has long been anathema to conservatives. As Alicia Mundy recently reported in an article in The Washington Monthly, the Koch brothers have funded a group called Concerned Veterans for America (CVA)—a veterans service organization (VSO) that has no veteran members and provides no veteran services.[19] Speaking about wait time problems, CVA CEO Pete Hegseth told a Koch brothers summit in 2014, "What you probably don't know is the central role that Concerned Veterans for America played in exposing and driving this [VA scandal] from the very beginning."[20]

This group is central to the Koch brothers' anti-government agenda and has been lobbying not only for partial and ultimately full privatization of the VHA but also against Obamacare and other government programs. In 2016 it launched a website. My VA Story, soliciting bad stories about the VHA from veterans. Needless to say, veterans with good stories about VHA care need not apply.

CVA has influenced the mainstream media narrative on the VHA, and newspapers, as well as TV and radio outlets, have been filled with stories about VHA dysfunction. This new media narrative has ignored continuing evidence that the VHA—in spite of wait-time delays and top-heavy management—continues to deliver high-quality care to veterans.

The fate of the VHA will affect more than America's 22 million veterans and their families. With its research, teaching, and innovative models of team-based integrated care, the VHA serves as a model for quality healthcare delivery that should be emulated rather than dismantled.[21]

CHAPTER THREE
THE NEW YORK TIMES WAIT-TIME FIXATION

IN HIS BOOK Best Care Anywhere, Phillip Longman provided a portrait of a healthcare delivery system for veterans (at least those who qualify for VHA services) that is far better than Medicare or private insurance. But most readers of the daily press would find Longman's picture at odds with the story of the VHA routinely depicted in the media. That's because of one recent overblown scandal combined with the Republican scapegoating of a fine public system that they underfund—and would love to privatize.

In February 2014 a VHA doctor in Phoenix, Arizona, blew the whistle on his own facility, where administrators had been falsifying records about the time it took for patients to see a doctor. These revelations about appointment delays, as reported in *The New York Times* and other media outlets, led to the resignation of then–Secretary of Veterans Affairs Eric Shinseki. President Barack Obama quickly appointed a replacement for him from the private sector, Robert A. McDonald, former CEO of Procter & Gamble.

In February 2014 Vermont Senator Bernie Sanders, then chairman of the Senate Committee on Veterans' Affairs, had asked for a $24-billion appropriation for the Department of Veterans Affairs (mostly for healthcare), which Senate Republicans blocked. After the Phoenix wait-time controversy was exposed, Sanders brokered a deal with Republican Senator John McCain, and Congress grudgingly gave the Department $16 billion—$8 billion less than requested. This kind of underfunding was guaranteed to lead to problems, not only because the VHA, in correcting its wait-time issues, has attracted many new enrollees, but also because of the nature of the veteran population the VHA serves. Nonetheless, McDonald changed VHA managerial practices, fired some administrators responsible for the Phoenix "scandal," and, most important, began recruiting much-needed new staff—particularly primary-care providers. By the end of 2016, the VHA had remedied many of its problems.

Despite the VHA's vigorous efforts to root out a localized management scam and, with far greater difficulty, remedy a shortage of primary-care providers that is nationwide in scope, congressional Republicans and many in the mainstream media continue to depict the VHA as being in a state of ongoing, almost terminal, crisis. *The New York Times*, for example, has published article after article depicting the VHA as a "troubled health system, especially in rural or out-of-the-way posts." According to the publication's multiple reports, sources are quoted over and over again attesting to the VHA's "corrosive culture" and the fact that it has lost the "trust" and "confidence" of its patients and has been rendered a "demoralized and dysfunctional agency." Even though one of its major stories challenged the contention that veterans had died because of wait times, the headline broadcast precisely the opposite: "V.A. Official Acknowledges Link between Delays and Patient Deaths."[22]

The Times continued its anti-VHA narrative in its coverage of veteran suicide by reporter Dave Phillips. In a 2015 article that filled two pages in the front section of the prestigious Sunday edition, Phillips focused on the high rate of suicides in the Second Marine Battalion, Seventh Regiment (2/7), deployed in the Helmand Province of Afghanistan for eight months in 2008. Both the veterans quoted in the article and its headline—"In Unit Stalked by Suicide, Veterans Try to Save One Another: Members of a Marine battalion that served in a restive region in Afghanistan have been devastated by the deaths of comrades and frustrated by the V.A."—placed the blame for veteran suicide directly on the VHA.[23] Nowhere did Phillips mention a study documenting that veterans treated at the VHA had lower suicide rates than those who did not seek help from the system.[24] When I emailed Phillips to ask him about his article, he replied, "I'm sorry I have to decline. I don't feel very qualified to speak. I'm not an expert, and generally speaking, what I know I have put in print."[25]

This kind of pack journalism has, not surprisingly, contributed to public views regarding the ability of the VA and the government to provide needed services. In November 2015 the Pew Research Center released a report on public perceptions of government. "Currently, just 19% say they can trust the government always or most of the time, among the lowest levels in the past half-century." As the report stated, the VA's problems took a "toll on its image." "Currently, just 39% view the VA favorably—a decline of 29 percentage points since October 2013, during the partial government shutdown."[26]

GETTING THE STORY RIGHT

The real VHA story is ideological opposition by the right—and clinical excellence despite chronic underfunding. The main opponents of the VHA are Republicans in Congress—the very legislators who go to great lengths to demonstrate their support for Americans in uniform. But when vets return home and are hidden from view, the right short-changes their care. During the Senate debate about the $24-billion Department of Veterans Affairs allocation, for example, then Alabama Senator Jeff Sessions echoed the sentiments of his fellow Republicans, insisting, "I don't think our veterans want their programs to be enhanced if every penny of the money to enhance those programs is added to the debt of the United States of America." Has he asked any vets about that? Moreover, politicians like Sessions take no responsibility for their policies, blaming the VHA for the predictable side effects.

The long-term Republican goal is to privatize the VHA, a policy that would cap costs, increase middleman profits, reduce the efficiencies of a fully integrated system, and drastically cut care. Only six months after Congress allocated funds devoted to increasing access to VHA services, the results of its own $8 billion shortfall were clear. Because of its successful efforts to provide more services to more veterans, the VHA was facing a budget gap and asking for another $2.5 billion. As Deputy Secretary of Veterans Affairs Sloan Gibson tried valiantly to explain at a June 25, 2015, hearing of the House Committee on Veterans' Affairs, the VHA has so successfully addressed wait-time problems that it had added 7 million more patient appointments and increased the number of patients receiving treatment, in some places by almost 20 percent. That success, obviously, increased costs.

But within the Republican caucus on both sides of Capitol Hill, this rise in costs was more proof of the VHA's dysfunction. House Speaker John Boehner of Ohio fulminated: "The VA's problem isn't funding—it's outright failure. Absolute failure to take care of our veterans." No injection of funds, he opined, can fix the department because it is just "a mess."[27]

Meanwhile, Florida Republican Jeff Miller, then chair of the House Veterans' Affairs Committee, accused the VHA of "a startling lack of transparency and accountability." On July 21, 2015, in an op-ed in the *Pittsburgh Post-Gazette*, Miller went even further, accusing the Department of Veterans Affairs of "years of mismanagement and a blatant lack of transparency and accountability. The department can't seem to meet any of its vital responsibilities—providing health care, approving disability benefits and constructing hospitals—without going billions over budget and falling years behind schedule."[28]

On July 22, 2015, McDonald appeared at another hearing before the House committee. He explained why the shortfall had reached $3 billion and suggested various ways to sort out some irrational practices that Congress had built into the VA budgeting practice, which gave Miller another opportunity to attack the system.

After these show-trial hearings, Congress gave the VHA a temporary budgetary reprieve by funding the shortfall. Even so, the new anti-VHA narrative, so popular with would-be GOP privatizers of the VHA, now dominates the public imagination.

When I tell my liberal and progressive friends that I am writing about

VHA healthcare, I invariably get some version of, "Oh, that must be so depressing." Can you blame them? Like many members of the media, most people don't understand how difficult it is to care for the very particular population of veterans the VHA actually serves. Moreover, few politicians and pundits understand or acknowledge that many of the problems the VHA faces reflect the skewed priorities of both our broader healthcare system and the institutions that educate its future professionals. Whereas the media and Republicans in Congress gleefully jump on any hint of problems at the VHA, news about its innovations in care rarely makes the headlines.

UNREPORTED SUCCESSES

Consider, for example, the results of the independent assessment mandated by the Choice Act and conducted by two nonprofit research companies, the RAND Corporation and the MITRE Corporation. When the assessment came out, there were virtually no press reports about its positive finding that the VHA consistently performs as well as and often better than private-sector healthcare providers.

Key findings of the report included:

- Postoperative morbidity was lower for VA patients compared with non-veterans receiving non-VA care.
- Inpatient care was as effective (or more so) in VA as in non-VA hospitals.
- VA hospitals were more likely to follow best practices in the use of central venous catheter line infection prevention, and rates of mortality declined more quickly in VA over time than in non-VA settings for specific conditions.

The report also found that veterans in nursing homes were less likely to develop pressure ulcers; outpatients and those suffering chronic conditions got better follow-up care; and VA health providers offered better mental health and obesity counseling and blood-pressure control, particularly for African-Americans. It is important to note that income and educational disparities were smaller at VHA facilities in such areas as diabetes, heart disease, and cancer screenings.

The report confirmed what many fighting for what is known as "right care"—defined as avoiding toxic, unnecessary tests, medications, and procedures—have long understood: that the VHA, contrary to its status as a

GOP and media whipping boy, has been a pioneer in providing clinically appropriate care to veterans.

Elderly patients in the VHA were less likely to receive the kinds of medications that can make them sicker and sometimes even kill them, the report found. VHA patients were more likely to be spared toxic chemotherapy within fourteen days of death or admitted to an ICU thirty days before death. This was attributed to the VHA's commitment to palliative and hospice care.[29]

Healthcare quality expert Charlene Harrington, professor emeritus at University of California, San Francisco, called the report "really impressive, particularly given the patient mix and chronic underfunding."

To be sure, the report also details a number of ways the VHA can improve—remedying chronic shortages of primary-care and specialist physicians in some areas of the country, dealing with lack of space in older VHA facilities, and repairing an aging information technology architecture.

The report also points to variation in treatment and quality in a system that has more than 150 hospitals and almost 1,000 community outpatient clinics. Here, however, it offers an important caveat: Variation in the private sector is sometimes even more pronounced. On some measures of care recommended to achieve clinical targets, the report found that "commercial HMOs, Medicare HMOs, and Medicaid HMOs all exhibited much more variability than the VA facilities."

Despite recent public criticism of the VA for long patient wait times, the study found the VA is actually performing well on this measure. To wit: "VA's reported wait times for new patient primary and specialty care are shorter than wait times reported in focused studies in the private sector." For those who live in rural areas short on VA facilities, the report added that "expanding access to non-VA providers may help with routine or emergency room care, but not with advanced or specialized care." Nor would veterans living in these areas have better access to teaching or academic facilities.

Months after the independent assessment appeared, another report from the RAND Corporation added more information—again unreported—about VHA care. The report, titled "Resources and Capabilities of the Department of Veterans Affairs to Provide Timely and Accessible Care to Veterans," noted that although there were differences in care and leadership culture across the system, researchers "did not find evidence of a systemwide crisis in access to VA care." In fact, the report identified congressional policies as one of the main barriers to VHA improvements (despite Veteran Affairs Committee Chairman Jeff Miller's apparent belief that firing VHA leaders is the solution to any access problems). The report noted that "inflexibility in budgeting stemming from the congressional appropriation processes," and concluded that the hastily designed and implemented Veterans Choice Program, "further complicated the situation and resulted in confusion among veterans, VA employees, and non-VA providers."[30]

Though it similarly received no media attention, another positive report on the VHA came from the Joint Commission, the independent nonprofit that accredits U.S. hospitals and healthcare organizations. After surveying the VHA between 2014 and 2015, the commission found improvements in access, timeliness, and coordination of care, as well as in leadership, safety, staffing, and competency.[31]

Every report on the VHA over the past two years has documented that the system provides care equal or superior to private-sector care and spotlighted significant improvements in problematic practices that led to two years of scandal-mongering on Capitol Hill and in the national media. But instead of lauding the VHA for its progress and working to sustain the system, federal lawmakers and critics are quick to jump on any hint of a glitch. The narrative of a dysfunctional VHA that the news media and some federal lawmakers promote does not acknowledge that the VHA is a national or global leader in fields like telemedicine, mental health, primary and geriatric care, and reducing opioid use. Instead, too many lawmakers lambast the VHA for not changing more rapidly, steadfastly ignoring the fact that changing the culture of any institution, particularly that of America's largest healthcare system, must take years. This, of course, is guaranteed to slowly cripple the VHA by making it harder to recruit needed staff. Why would physicians, nurse-practitioners, social workers, psychologists, and other professionals want to work in a system depicted as broken beyond repair, doomed to disappear, and filled with demoralized staff?[32]

CHAPTER FOUR
BERNIE SANDERS AND THE VHA

ON THE FRONT PAGE OF ITS Sunday edition on February 7, 2016, *The New York Times* published a wildly misleading story titled, "Faith in Agency Clouded Bernie Sanders's V.A. Response," written by Steve Eder and Dave Phillips.[33]

The gist of the piece was that Sanders, blinded by his friendliness to government agencies, did not acknowledge the VA scandal of long wait times for services until very late in the game. But if you read far enough into the detail of the story, you find that the allegation made in the headline is not documented at all—quite the opposite is true.

As the *Times* admitted much later in the piece, Sanders, as chairman of the Committee on Veterans' Affairs, realized that Republicans were seriously underfunding the VA and fought hard for adequate financing. It was the underfunding, not the deeply flawed agency imagined by the *Times*, that led to the long wait times.

The Times got the story wrong in its earlier reporting of this trumped-up scandal, and its attack on Sanders relied on its earlier mistakes. For nearly two years, its reporters have been shaping and amplifying a deeply flawed and factually challenged mainstream media narrative that dovetails neatly with the privatizing agenda of right-wing Republicans in Washington.

In actual fact, the VHA is far more cost-effective and compassionate than other counterparts in the healthcare system treating comparable patients. The right's agenda, a threat that Sanders appreciated early on, is to privatize much of the VHA. Wade Miller, a Heritage Foundation–funded critic of the VHA, expressed the GOP bias well when he argued that "The best way we can help veterans is by reducing their need to use the VA." According to Miller, the "biggest hurdle" to meeting that increased demand is the very fact that veterans' healthcare is provided by "a government program."[34]

In the story by Eder and Phillips, the *Times* revisited congressional debates about VHA funding and service delivery in 2014 that were much influenced by this perspective. However, the GOP's ideological fixation with shrinking government is cited only in passing, via a single reference to the views of "some Republican Presidential candidates and a veterans' organization backed by the billionaires Charles G. and David H. Koch."

Instead, Eder and Phillips focused their criticism on Sanders. When Republican opposition to measures like SB 1982, a $21-billion funding package that Sanders introduced in early 2014, helped aggravate the longer wait times that became a *Times*-reported "scandal" later that same year, Sanders faced "a moment of crisis," according to Eder and Phillips. "His deep-seated faith in the fundamental goodness of government blinded him, at least at first, to a dangerous breakdown in the one corner of it he was supposed to police."

What was slowing Sanders down and revealing supposed leadership shortcomings, then and now? In part, the *Times* contends, it was because he "initially saw a conservative plot" to discredit and undermine the VHA so more veterans would support dismantling of the VHA and its replacement with private-sector healthcare coverage instead. Was this threat a mere figment of the senator's imagination? Apparently not, according to his rival for the Democratic presidential nomination. Just three days before the *Times* piece debunking Sanders' defense of the VHA appeared, Hillary Clinton told MSNBC debate viewers the push for VHA privatization is "another part of the Koch brothers' agenda. They've actually formed an organization to try to convince Americans we should no longer have guaranteed health care, specialized health care for our veterans." Like Sanders—and under pressure from him on this issue—Clinton said she would work with other "veterans' service organizations, the veterans of America" to "fix the V.A." but would "never let it be privatized."

The group Clinton was referring to is CV A, which has few actual members, and unlike real VSOs—like the Disabled American Veterans (DAV), Veterans of Foreign Wars (VFW), Paralyzed Veterans of America, and Amvets—it provides no services to veterans. Until only six months ago, these four traditional VSOs worked in an alliance called the Independent Budget. In the past this coalition provided Congress and the White House with its own assessment of the VA's funding needs. Sanders consulted all of those groups when crafting SB 1982, and they supported it.

The other veterans' group the *Times* reporters quoted heavily is Iraq and Afghanistan Veterans of America (IAVA). According to a monograph by Stephen Trynosky on the political environment that now influences the fate of the VHA, the IAVA is a new kind of VSO—one that has "assiduously embraced a fundraising and revenue model focused heavily on corporate underwriting...The group's 2012 annual report lists a constellation of corporate donors and wealthy patrons, some of whom appear to have an interest in the increased privatization of VHA services."[35]

The Times presented the $21-billion price tag for SB 1982 as excessive, when $21 billion spent over ten years is just a sliver of the VA's total annual budget of about $160 billion, and minuscule compared to the more than a trillion dollars in direct spending on the Iraq and Afghanistan wars that have created so much demand for VHA services. As the *Times* acknowledged late in the piece, Sanders did work effectively with his Republican counterparts to enact a $16-billion bill—less than was needed but enough to finance improvements. So apparently, the $21 billion that Sanders originally called for wasn't so crazy.

In short, Sanders saw the privatization threat and the consequences of underfunding well in advance. He did his best to deal with both threats but was blocked by Republicans. As the Times also admitted toward the end of the article, Sanders' original $21-billion funding bill actually got 56 votes in the Senate—not a fringe measure at all—but was blocked by a filibuster. In fact, Republican opponents of the bill weren't "puzzled" by it as the *Times* reports—they were adamant that more money should not be spent on veterans' healthcare—unless that money was channeled, through the Choice Act and other Republican-sponsored legislative proposals, to private-sector providers. Judging by the facts of the case, a better headline and storyline for the piece could have been, "Sanders Resisted GOP Assault on Veterans' Benefits."

The Times needs to move its singular fixation on wait times—real or exaggerated—and also inform its readers about the things the VA does well. A recent study, for example, compared the outcomes for 700,000 California cancer patients who were treated at the VHA with patients covered by private insurance or Medicare and Medicaid. Particularly relevant to the current wait-time debate, it documents the fact that although veterans had to wait longer for access to care than those covered by the other insurance programs, they received more appropriate treatment and had better outcomes.[36] As one of its authors, Kenneth W. Kizer, MD, MPH (and former undersecretary for health at the VA), explains, short delays in care, although unacceptable, may not be as important a variable as getting the right kind of care, which is why, according to Garry Augustine, executive director of the DAV, most of his 1.3 million members want delays in care to be fixed and the system to be well funded because they "prefer to be treated at the VHA where they receive holistic services in one place instead of the kind of disjointed care they get in the private sector."[37]

CHAPTER FIVE:
WITH FRIENDS LIKE THESE

SENATOR JOHN MCCAIN WORKED with Senator Bernie Sanders to craft the veterans' healthcare bill now known as the Choice Act in 2014, which allowed veterans facing long wait times or living more than forty miles from the nearest VHA facility to get coverage in the private sector. Though it was only a three-year pilot program, the Arizona Republican immediately set out to renege on his promise that the Choice Act would be temporary and began floating plans to make it permanent.

Throughout 2015 and 2016, McCain lobbied hard for a bill that would eliminate any restrictions on veterans' access to private-sector healthcare. McCain's gift to veterans is a bill misleadingly labeled The Care They Deserve Act. It would make the Choice Act permanent.

Under McCain's new plan, the nine million veterans eligible for VHA care would be free to use any private healthcare facility or provider, for any form of service, with the federal government paying the tab—no questions asked. McCain gathered seven other Republican sponsors for his bill, all of them pushing the new conservative narrative that the VHA is broken beyond repair. This push ignores reports by a Choice Act–mandated independent assessment of the VHA, which documents that its veteran patients actually receive better care, at lower cost, than millions of Americans who rely on private-sector healthcare.

What's wrong with The Care They Deserve Act? Just about everything, which is why many VSOs like DAV and Vietnam Veterans of America oppose the plan, and why the VHA's own undersecretary for health, David Shulkin, has proposed a more sensible alternative.

Economists who advised the Commission on Care estimated that McCain-style privatization could triple the cost of veterans' care to almost $450 billion a year—money that would not be well spent. The VHA's clinicians and other staff specialize in the complex health problems related to military service and deal with patients who are older, sicker, poorer, and with more mental health problems than those cared for in the private sector. The average elderly patient in the private sector shows up presenting between three to five physical problems. The "co-morbidities" of a Vietnam vet, for example, can number from 9 to 12. That's why VHA primary-care providers spend at least thirty minutes with their patients per visit, compared to the ten or fifteen minutes allotted to patients in the private sector. Will private-sector providers want to take the time to care for aging, sometimes homeless, often mentally ill, veterans? Even if they do, will they be able to detect the difference between ordinary Type 2 and Agent Orange–related diabetes or be equipped to parse the myriad symptoms of PTSD?

In 2014 RAND conducted a study comparing VA mental and behavioral health programs with those in the private sector. To find out whether private-sector providers were, in fact, "Ready to Serve" the nation's veterans, the study focused on two common problems from which veterans suffer—PTSD and major depressive disorder (MDD). The study documented that the vast majority of VHA mental health providers (70 percent) had the knowledge of service-related problems—what is known as military cultural competency—necessary to assess and treat veterans. When it came to private-sector therapists in the TRICARE network, the score dropped precipitously—to 24 percent—and plummeted even further—to 8 percent—for those private-sector mental health providers with no military or TRICARE affiliation.[38]

In a startling finding, RAND documented that only 30 percent of private-sector clinicians (including social workers, psychologists, and psychiatrists) reported using evidence-based therapies to treat their private-sector patients who suffered from PTSD and MDD, compared with 75 percent of VHA clinicians who used evidence-based practices.[39]

Ignoring such highly publicized evidence, McCain's bill is built on several erroneous assumptions. One is that private-sector care is always better than that delivered by the public sector. The second is that giving veterans unrestricted choice between VHA and private-sector healthcare will not erode the veterans' health system. In reality the Choice bill would ultimately erode real choice by weakening the VHA option, putting the entire veterans' health system at risk. The VHA's current budget is, in part, determined by how many veterans use the system and for what services. If far more eligible veterans start using private-sector healthcare, there will be less funding available for VHA services that are unavailable elsewhere and for maintaining the agency's highly specialized research and clinical expertise in military-related health problems. As funding for costly private-sector care eats up more of the VHA's annual budget, there will be hospital and clinic closings, along with VHA staff layoffs. To reduce expenditures on veteran healthcare, Congress may also be tempted to make eligibility for benefits even more restrictive than it is today.[40]

CHAPTER SIX
WHAT KIND OF PATIENT EXPERIENCE?

WHEN HE WAS VA SECRETARY neither Bob McDonald nor the VHA he oversaw ever seemed to catch a break. On May 23, 2016, a reporter questioned McDonald about the VHA's tracking of patient appointment times around the country. McDonald's predecessor was forced to quit over allegations of appointment delays and a cover-up at a Phoenix VHA hospital, and McDonald has often been on the defensive about the issue as the agency tries to hire the additional caregivers needed for the influx of Iraq and Afghanistan veterans.

In his response to the reporter, McDonald suggested that, in the meantime, the VHA's performance should be judged by a broader set of metrics. "What really counts is how does the veteran feel about their encounter with the VA?" McDonald said. "When you go to Disney, do they measure the number of hours you wait in line? What is important is your satisfaction with the experience."[41]

Unfortunately for the secretary, his invocation of the Magic Kingdom triggered a pack-journalism social-media response. CVA immediately denounced McDonald on its website, claiming he showed disrespect for all VHA patients: "The sacrifice that accompanies earning that care is not the same as the sacrifice of taking a road trip to Florida," the CVA declared. "Shame on Bob McDonald for trivializing veteran wait times this way."[42]

House Speaker Paul Ryan called the remark "disgusting" and "beyond the pale," a sentiment shared by House Veterans' Affairs Committee Chair

Jeff Miller, a frequent critic of McDonald and ally of CVA in seeking to dismantle and privatize the VHA. There was even talk of calling for McDonald's resignation.[43]

After two days of negative news coverage, McDonald, a veteran himself, issued a clarification and apology to any veteran who felt his comments trivialized the VHA's "noble mission."[44] But lost in the Republican baying for more blood was a great political irony: Throughout private-sector healthcare, Disney's corporate model for gauging customer satisfaction is now widely used to determine patient satisfaction and to regulate the patient experience.

Quality patient care requires an application of skills, experience, and teamwork quite different from the prerequisites for good customer service in the hospitality or entertainment industries. Yet treating sick people as "customers" has become part of mainstream management thinking.

The Disneyfication trend took off ten years ago after consultant Fred Lee published the bestselling *If Disney Ran Your Hospital: 9 1/2 Things You Would Do Differently*. Patient surveys using methods and metrics from resort hotels and amusement parks are now the norm in U.S. healthcare.[45] A hospital's results on the Hospital Consumer Assessment of Health Care Providers and Systems (HCAHCPS) standardized survey even determine, in part, its reimbursement rate for federally subsidized patients.[46]

Disneyfication has spawned a huge crowd of high-priced consultants, like Lee and Quint Studer of the Studer Group, who teach hospitals how to improve their patient-qua-customer experience to score well on questionnaires. As Studer puts it in his *HCAHCPS Handbook*, hospital administrators need to "manage the patient's expectations" to succeed by convincing patients they are receiving good personal care—even if the hospital has poor nurse–patient ratios or lousy patient safety records.[47]

In some hospitals, nursing staff that are trained and managed under this model have been forced to use scripts when interacting with patients and families. They are coached to smile and repeat words and phrases (such as "excellent care") that administrators want to see echoed in patient surveys.

Some hospitals now designate an employee to be "chief patient experience officer" (CXO), a position enjoying executive status. As CEO of the Cleveland Clinic, Delos "Toby" Cosgrove, vice chairman of the VA Commission on Care, has overseen annual patient experience conferences for the past eight years. Despite having both a CXO and a patient experience office, the Cleveland Clinic has been investigated for patient safety lapses that almost resulted in the hospital's suspension from the Medicare program.[48] Some suspect Cosgrove withdrew his name for consideration as VA secretary because confirmation hearings would have led to negative publicity for the clinic.

Inappropriately treating—and, in fact, trivializing—sick patients as customers is a central feature of healthcare corporatization and represents everything the VHA has never been and should not become. If it's not good for veterans, it shouldn't be good for any of us. But that would mean critics of the VHA would have to apply the same standard to the government agency as they do to private-sector healthcare.[49]

CHAPTER SEVEN
IN DEFENSE OF ART

THE VHA HAS TAKEN A lot of heat in the past couple of years about using money to purchase art for its hospitals and other facilities. On September 8, 2016, Gail Collins, in a column in *The New York Times*, joined in the pile-on. Although Collins defended the VHA and opposed its privatization, writing that veterans "are satisfied" with its services and that "the care is in many cases excellent," she couldn't resist a jab at the VHA for spending $670,000 on two sculptures that were placed in a blind rehabilitation center. Her conclusion? "Veterans healthcare for everybody! But maybe with less art." When I checked *The New York Times* for footnoting purposes, the online story had no offending references to VA art, and the article contained no mention of the high-quality, cost-effective care the VHA delivers.[50] Absent a hard copy of The New York Times from September 8, 2016, the only way to find Collins' original article is to search newspapers that carried the syndicated column, for example, the *Seattle Times*.[51]

The issue of spending on art first emerged in 2015 when Congressman Jeff Miller (R—Fla.), Chairman of the House Veterans' Affairs Committee and a staunch advocate of VHA privatization, lambasted the VHA for spending $483,000 for a sculpture in a hospital courtyard. For Miller, whom Donald Trump promised to appoint to the post of secretary of veterans affairs if he was elected, the issue was not the quality of the art used at VHA facilities but the fact that the VHA was using taxpayer money on art, period. Miller called such spending "wanton and abusive."[52]

Miller's critique was faithfully broadcast by the mainstream media. As usual, reporters ignored several crucial facts, notably, how much of the budget such spending represents and the medical utility of art in hospitals and other healthcare facilities.

Between 2010 and 2016, the VHA has spent $5.4 million on commissioned artwork for over 1,500 facilities. This sum represents an infinitesimal sliver of the VHA's budget over that same period. The $483,000 Miller highlighted is, for example, 0.000007 percent of the VHA's $65-billion budget in 2017. But what is perhaps most disturbing about this focus on VHA art is its failure to understand why the VHA uses art in its hospitals and other facilities as well as the double messages the media and Congress send to VHA leaders, employees, and veterans themselves.

The VHA uses art in places like the newly constructed facility in Las Vegas, which commissioned several soothing water sculptures to help allay the anxiety of veterans with mental and physical illnesses as they wait for appointments. It is used to conceal medical equipment in hospices that care for dying veterans, in nursing homes where aging veterans will live out their lives, and in medical facilities like the Blind Rehabilitation Centers Collins mentions in her column. In fact, most of the veterans served in such rehabilitation facilities are not totally blind but rather visually impaired. They can, in fact, see the sculptures she complained about, as can their family and friends and the staff who care for them.

VHA facilities use art because scientific research has documented that art enhances patient healing and can even reduce hospital stays and thus save money.[53] This use of art is widely promoted in private-sector hospitals. The National Institute of Biotechnology Information website, for example, displays a peer-reviewed article on the Cleveland Clinic's art collection, lauding its positive use of art in medicine. "Fine art is good medicine. It comforts, elevates the spirit, and affirms life and hope," author Jennifer Finkel notes.[54]

The *Wall Street Journal* similarly praised the use of art in private-sector hospitals.[55] One of the hospitals highlighted for its pioneering work in the field was again the Cleveland Clinic and its use of the work of the Spanish artist Jaume Plensa, whose works sell for a princely sum.

The Cleveland Clinic, whose CEO Toby Cosgrove served as the vice chairman of the VA Commission on Care, proudly advertises its arts program on its websites. "The mission of the Cleveland Clinic Art Program is to enrich, inspire and enliven our patients, visitors, employees and community and to embody the core values of the institution: collaboration, quality, integrity, compassion, and commitment."[56] The website offers a virtual tour of its permanent—and very expensive—collection.

The Henry Ford Health System, whose CEO Nancy Schlichting served as chair of the VA Commission on Care, also boasts about its Healing Arts.[57] Any art used in private-sector hospitals is also purchased with the help of taxpayer money in the form of Medicare and Medicaid payments to those institutions. As far as can be documented, neither the Cleveland Clinic, Henry Ford Health System, or any other private-sector hospital has ever been asked to shut down its art exhibits because of the misuse of taxpayer dollars.

Quite the contrary. On September 8, 2016, when both Schlichting and Cosgrove appeared at the House Veterans' Affairs Committee meeting on the commission report regarding the future of the VHA, they received nothing but respectful comments from Miller and other committee members. In fact, both institutions were held up as precisely the kind of healthcare system veterans deserve and that the VHA should emulate.

There is a lot of talk about failures in leadership at the VHA, and surely there are many. But what kind of messages and guidance do VHA executives receive from their congressional overseers and media watchdogs? They are asked to emulate the private sector, which can apparently do no wrong, but when the VHA either leads or follow practices in the private sector, it is castigated for its efforts.

Art, anyone?[58]

SECTION TWO

CONGRESS AND THE COMMISSION

AS PART OF THE VETERANS ACCESS, Choice, and Accountability Act of 2014, Congress created a Commission on Care, "charging it to examine veterans' access to Department of Veterans Affairs health care and to examine strategically how best to organize the Veterans Health Administration, locate health resources, and deliver health care to veterans during the next 20 years."[59] The fifteen-member commission began holding meetings in 2015. Some of these meetings were behind closed doors; others were open to the public. The commission was supposed to issue a final report in 2015. Unable to finish its deliberations, it issued an interim report in December 2015. It issued its final report in August 2016.

The commission's members were chosen on partisan grounds. The House speaker and Senate majority leaders chose three members each. Six (three each) were chosen by the House and Senate minority leaders, and three by the White House. From the beginning the commission was stacked with a majority of members who were either downright hostile to or skeptical about the VHA. Even some Democratic picks were either unfamiliar with the VHA or supporters of market-based healthcare for veterans. Rear Admiral Joyce Johnson, a White House pick, had helped move the provision of healthcare out of the Coast Guard and into the private sector. She turned out to be a champion of total VHA privatization. Although Chair Nancy Schlichting was more supportive of the VHA, as CEO of the Henry Ford Health System, her institution had a great deal to gain from channeling veterans into the private sector. Vice Chair Toby Cosgrove, CEO of the Cleveland Clinic, was an outspoken champion of privatization, as was hospital CEO David Blom and hospital executive Marshall Webster. Another commissioner was Stewart M. Hickey, a former leader of Amvets, a group that broke away from a coalition of large VSOs because of its support for the CVA agenda.

All four were part of a rump group—the Strawman group—of commissioners favoring privatization. Another member of this group was Darin Selnick, a paid consultant with the Koch brothers–funded CVA, who dissented from the commission's final report, which, in his view, did not do enough to move veterans into private-sector healthcare. The only members of the commission who understood and supported not only saving but strengthening the VHA were Phillip Longman, author of B*est Care Anywhere*; Michael Blecker, a Vietnam veteran and executive of the San Francisco–based veterans' organization Swords to Plowshares; and David Gorman, a disabled Vietnam veteran and executive director of the DAV National Service and Legislative Headquarters in Washington, D.C. It was thus no surprise that its deliberations were marked by controversy, a failure to listen to the voices of many veterans, and unprecedented congressional attempts to compromise its tenuous independence.

CHAPTER EIGHT
CHAIRMAN MILLER INTERFERES

ON MARCH 14, 2016, Republican Congressman Jeff Miller, the House Veterans' Affairs Committee chairman and a staunch advocate of privatizing the VHA, wrote an angry letter to Commission Chair Nancy Schlichting.[60] In this unprecedented missive, Miller personally attacked Phillip Longman, a commission member who has advocated for not only preserving but strengthening the veterans' healthcare agency, in part by eliminating its cumbersome eligibility requirements and expanding healthcare services to veterans' families.

Miller accused Longman, a *Washington Monthly* senior editor, of personally editing a recent article by former *Wall Street Journal* reporter Alicia Mundy.[61] Mundy criticized Miller for his singular focus on VHA wait times and his insistence that forty veterans had died because they were waiting for care. She also detailed the role that Miller and other congressional conservatives have played in the Koch brothers' campaign to privatize veterans' healthcare. Mundy warned that private hospital systems, which have representatives on the commission, are "circling like vultures over the idea of dividing up the VA's multibillion-dollar budget."

Miller said Longman helped spread "blatantly false propaganda in an attempt to minimize the wait-times scandal at the Department of Veterans Affairs" through the Mundy magazine article. Longman "either believes the article's false claims or he—as an editor of the piece—signed off on them knowing they were untrue," Miller wrote. He warned the commissioners "to take anything Longman says with an extremely large grain of salt."

A subsequent *Washington Monthly* blog post by Paul Glastris, who actually edited Mundy's article, rebutted Miller's claims about patient deaths and other issues.[62] Longman, who is a part-time staff member at the magazine, also reviewed Mundy's piece but did not edit it. (Incidentally, members on the commission were permitted to continue to perform their professional duties as long as they did not claim to be acting on behalf of or speaking for the commission.)

Veterans' advocates say that Miller's tirade was the first time any of them could remember a member of Congress attacking a commissioner. Retired Army Captain Steve Robertson, a former Senate Veterans' Affairs Committee staff director, said that, in his thirty years working on veterans' issues, he couldn't "recall a member of Congress ever instructing members of a commission or advisory group to ignore one of their members." Robertson said, "Miller is way out of line." Another representative of a major VSO, who did not wish to be identified, called Miller's letter an attempt to "intimidate an independent commission and politicize their recommendations."

One week later Miller appeared before the commission and continued his critique of the agency. In his hourlong commentary, Miller had nothing good to say about the VHA. He ignored the findings of an independent assessment commissioned by Congress that found that the VHA delivers care that is often superior to that in the private sector. When commission member Michael Blecker tried to defend the VHA's model of integrated care and worried that many veterans would fall through the cracks of a private healthcare system, Miller barely let Blecker finish his comments. The congressman argued that the VHA is "holding veterans inside" the system and must allow them to move into private-sector care. Miller concluded by encouraging the commission to offer "bold ideas" on overhauling the system in their upcoming report.[63]

The congressman may indeed want to "empower veterans," as he termed it. But moving them into a private healthcare sector that has primary-care physician shortages, coordination of care difficulties, serious wait-time challenges, and hundreds of thousands of deaths from preventable medical errors poses risks that cannot be ignored.[64]

CHAPTER NINE
THE STRAWMAN DOCUMENT

DELIBERATIONS BY THE DEPARTMENT of Veterans Affairs Commission on Care, the congressionally mandated group planning the future of the VHA, were consistently marred by controversy. At a meeting of the commission in Washington in mid-March of 2016, a furor erupted when a proposal to privatize the VHA set off a firestorm of protest within the veterans' community.

Just before the meeting, several members of the commission learned that seven of their colleagues had been secretly gathering to draft a proposal to totally eliminate the VHA by 2035 and turn its taxpayer-funded functions over to the private sector. Those commissioners dubbed the plan "The Strawman Document."[65]

The authors of the Strawman Document insisted that the VHA is so "seriously broken" that "there is no efficient path to repair it." Although the commission's work was supposed to be data-driven and done by all the commissioners together, the faction meeting independently ignored many of the studies that indicated that treatment at the VHA is often better and more cost-effective than the care available in the private sector.[66]

It was not surprising that the Strawman group chose to ignore this research; its members had a vested interest in dismantling the VHA. The Strawman authors include Darin S. Selnick of the CVA and Stewart M. Hickey, a former leader of Amvets.

The Strawman authors acknowledged that private-sector healthcare systems do not provide integrated care, high-quality mental health treatment, or many other specialized services that the VHA currently delivers. But if the VHA became an insurer—paying the bills instead of providing direct care—it could spend more money trying to "incentivize" providers to give better care in these areas, they claimed.

Private hospitals would also get federal funding to run what are now VHA Centers of Excellence, which treat epilepsy, Parkinson's disease, and other conditions veterans face.

Representatives of several VSOs believed the secret meetings of the Strawman group may have violated the Sunshine and Federal Advisory Committee Acts, as well as the commission's agreed-upon processes.

The commission had set up working groups to consider key VHA issues. Unlike the secret Strawman meetings, subcommittee activities were well known to all members and the public. Meeting times were posted, and discussion minutes were recorded.

The Strawman faction engaged in another end run around their colleagues when they met with Republican Representative Jeff Miller, chair of the House Veterans' Affairs Committee, and Speaker Paul Ryan. One representative of a major VSO, who asked not to be identified, observed: "If the authors requested the meeting with the House leadership, that constitutes lobbying. If they were invited by the House leadership, that constitutes more interference into the commission's deliberations. Either way, this meeting, funded by the U.S. taxpayer, was totally inappropriate."

"The plan does represent a complete deflection of responsibility to subject these men and women to an alternative 'payer-only' system of care that not only is ill-equipped to absorb the demand but is also, at best, minimally equipped in terms of expertise and the ability to coordinate such complex care over a veteran's lifetime," said Sherman Gillums Jr., acting executive director of Paralyzed Veterans of America.

Before the Strawman proposal became public, DAV launched Setting the Record Straight—a social media campaign against proposals that would privatize some or all of the VHA.[67] Garry Augustine, DAV's Washington executive director, said: "Although we have voiced our views about VA health care for the future, it seems many on the commission are committed to [doing] away with the VA health care system and turn veterans over to private health care, which we believe would result in uncoordinated and fragmented care for veterans."

The commission would have done far better to consider the views of VA Undersecretary of Health David Shulkin and commission member Phillip Longman.[68] Shulkin has argued for strengthening the VHA and giving it a more active role in directing and coordinating any care veterans receive in the private-sector system. Longman believes that the VHA should serve all veterans—not just those with service-related conditions or those who are low-income.[69]

CHAPTER TEN
THE COMMISSION'S FINAL REPORT

AFTER ALMOST A YEAR OF meetings and hearings, the Commission on Care issued its report on the future of the VHA on June 30, 2016. "Care delivered by the VA," the report states, "is in many ways comparable or better in clinical quality to that generally available in the private sector."[70]

But with problems in accessing services, variations in care, and the managerial culture at various facilities, the commission argued that the major remedy was not outright privatization but in giving veterans more private-sector options, a finding that veterans' groups fear may also weaken the decades-old system.

One of the commission's most complex and potentially problematic recommendations involves the creation of a "VHA Care System" that would integrate private-sector providers into a VHA-supervised network. The network would service only those veterans eligible for VHA services. Currently, about nine million veterans have been able to establish VHA eligibility; that is, they have health problems connected to their military service or a low-enough income to qualify for enrollment.

The commission recommended that veterans who are VHA-eligible would choose a primary-care provider who, in turn, would refer them to specialists. These primary-care doctors or specialists could work within the VHA or go outside the VHA to be providers who contract with the agency.

The VHA would be required to create a network that includes all providers who take care of veterans. The agency would have to screen and then contract with community or private-sector providers and ensure that those providers use information technology systems that are compatible with the VHA's networks. The VHA would also have to make sure that those providers understand military culture and would be responsible for coordinating the care veterans receive and helping them navigate the system.

Working with the private sector to coordinate veterans' care will not be easy. The commission found that veterans who are treated in the VHA receive coordinated care, whereas those with private plans, Medicare, or TRICARE receive care that is of "lower quality, threatens patient safety, and shifts costs among payers."

The commission also suggested revising the byzantine VA eligibility requirements that deny benefits to veterans who were "dismissed from military service with an other-than-honorable discharge because of actions that resulted from health conditions (such as traumatic brain injury, post-traumatic stress disorder, or substance use) caused by, or exacerbated by, their service."

According to the report, the VHA also needs more funding for competitive salaries, which will help with recruitment and retention of professional staff. As there are nationwide shortages of certain healthcare professionals, recruiting will not be easy.

The commission estimated that over the next few decades, about 40 to 60 percent of veterans will receive some, if not all, of their healthcare from private-sector providers. Treating fewer patients could significantly compromise VHA care if healthcare providers cannot maintain their clinical skills. Those developments could also discourage healthcare professionals from working in or staying with the VHA, which could lead to closing some facilities. "Reductions in volume of care within VA facilities, and potentially adverse effects on quality" are not addressed, the report noted.

The commission's recommendations are a product of a political fracture within the commission itself. Members who supported the VHA constantly fought with hospital-industry executives as well as representatives of the conservative Koch brothers–funded CVA, the so-called Strawman group, which advocated dismantling VHA. Darin Selnick and Stewart Hickey, commissioners who were both connected to CVA, refused to sign the final report. They viewed it as weak on privatization.[71]

Two other commissioners had differing views. Michael Blecker, a Vietnam veteran and executive director of Swords to Plowshares, a San Francisco–based veterans' organization, refused to sign the document because of serious concerns that the proposed healthcare system "would threaten the viability of VA care for millions of veterans who rely on it." He expressed his concerns in an eloquent letter of dissent sent to the commission.[72] However, Phillip Longman supported the plan with some reservations. He believes it could bring more veterans into the VHA system and improve the quality of care.

To provide a stronger system, Congress would have to allocate more funds to allow the VHA to hire the necessary staff to provide direct care and handle all the demands of integrating private-sector contractors into the veterans' healthcare system. Without these resources, the integrity of the VHA will be compromised, and the agency would face blame for poor care that veterans receive.

There is little indication that conservatives would provide the resources and time necessary to engage in the truly herculean task of creating a VHA health system that coordinates care with the private sector. The VHA privatization bills proposed by Senator John McCain, an Arizona Republican, and Representative Cathy McMorris Rodgers, a Washington Republican (supported by Representative Jeff Miller, a Florida Republican and chair of the House Veterans' Affairs Committee), obviously would starve the agency, not support it.[73] One of Donald Trump's proposals to give all veterans vouchers for use in the private sector would effectively eliminate the VHA. Trump announced this plan while running for president, and it sparked outrage from veterans' groups and unions.

Representatives of VF W, the American Legion, DAV, I A V A, Vietnam Veterans of America, Paralyzed Veterans of America, Got Your Six, and Military Officers Association of America have adamantly rejected the dismantling of the VHA. Many privatization schemes, they warned, would lead to higher costs and, the VSOs fear, even more limitations on access to services. Veterans with complex physical and mental conditions would receive no care coordination from the VHA, which, given the reality of private-sector healthcare, would mean no care coordination at all.

As Rick Weidman, executive director for government and policy affairs at Vietnam Veterans of America, explained, care coordination is critical because veterans have far more complex problems than the average private-sector patient, which is why Weidman also urged commissioners to move beyond anonymous data when estimating future VHA use. Yes, the number of veterans the VHA serves will diminish as World War II, Korean, and Vietnam War veterans die. The veterans who still use the VHA, however, will be sicker than the average private-sector patient.

Seven of the VSO leaders wrote a letter to the commission, making it completely clear what they and their members want: "the development of local integrated community networks in which VA serves as the coordinator and primary provider of health care to veterans; non-VA community care would be integrated into this network to fill gaps and expand access."[74]

A number of other groups also responded strongly to the commission's final report. The Association of VA Psychology Leaders, the Association of VA Social Workers, and unions representing VA employees issued a policy brief opposing the Commission on Care's proposal to create a new VHA care system, which would ultimately channel up to 60 percent of eligible veterans into private-sector healthcare. Two independent national groups, the American Psychological Association (APA) and the National Association of Social Workers, also signed the policy paper.[75]

In an email, Heather O'Beirne Kelly, the APA's lead psychologist on military and veterans policy, told me that the APA "is opposed to the primary recommendation of the Commission on Care's report, which we feel would in effect disassemble one of the most successful, innovative features of current VA care: the primary care/mental health integrated approach."

VSOs, professional associations, and interested citizens are not the only ones who will influence the future of the VHA. As we have seen, the nation's media have already played a role in shaping the new VHA narrative. Mainstream media outlets like CNN that use headlines like "Billions spent to fix VA didn't solve problems, made some issues worse" to describe the commission report help create a "VHA is broken beyond repair" narrative.[76] Although *The New York Times* has been extremely critical of the VHA, its July 2016 editorial opposing VHA privatization could turn what many veterans groups see as an anti-VHA bent in the national news media.[77]

It is ironic that the commission report stressed that the VHA currently delivers some of the best care anywhere. Rather than just talking about teamwork, most VHA providers actually work in teams, communicate with one another on electronic medical records, and help patients avoid unnecessary and dangerous overtreatment. The VHA also provides some of the best services for mental health, rehabilitation, and homelessness in the country.

A plan that contributes to strengthening the VHA and improving the private-sector healthcare system would be a positive development for veterans and all the rest of us. But if the deficiencies in the civilian healthcare system begin to infect the VHA, millions of Americans will lose out.[78]

CHAPTER ELEVEN
NOT EVERYONE HEARD ON CAPITOL HILL

WHEN THE HOUSE VETERANS' Affairs Committee held a hearing on the final recommendations of the VA Commission on Care on September 7, 2016, not a single VSO was asked to speak, in spite of the fact that such groups represent millions of former military personnel.

Also noticeably absent was Vietnam veteran Michael Blecker, executive director of Swords to Plowshares, who served on the Commission on Care and dissented from its final report. Blecker objected that the commission's leading recommendation—the creation of a so-called VHA health system network of private-sector providers. Blecker, who says he is not opposed to some expansion of the use of outside physicians or hospitals under limited circumstances, argued that channeling more veterans into the private sector would deprive the VHA of the patient base it needs to continue operating, fragment specialists from primary care, and thus "threaten the viability of VA care for millions of veterans who rely on it...That is not a veteran health care system worth serving for."[79]

Instead, Committee Chair Jeff Miller invited only two people to testify before the panel: Cosgrove and Schlichting. Miller was a faithful supporter of Donald Trump, who, while he was campaigning for president, touted the VA committee's chairman as his top pick as secretary of veterans' affairs in any Trump administration. (Miller was opposed by many veterans' groups and passed over by Trump when he won the election).

Although Schlichting expressed support for the VHA, Cosgrove was one of the leaders of the Straw Man group. Cosgrove and Schlichting both expressed enthusiasm for creating a VHA care system that ostensibly would create a network of private-sector providers to deliver healthcare to veterans while also somehow integrating them into the VHA. The report estimated that this system would eventually channel up to 60 percent of veterans into private-sector healthcare and even acknowledges that the new setup would potentially weaken the VHA itself.

It is alarming that all the Democrats on the committee—with one notable exception—voiced support for this general policy direction, albeit with less ideological fervor than Miller and his GOP colleagues. The one committee member who spoke out against the plan—fortunately for veterans—was ranking Democrat James Takano of California, who expressed serious reservations about the proposed VHA care system and echoed concerns about it that had already been raised by President Obama and VA Secretary MacDonald.

Some other Democrats came across as shockingly misinformed. Some, for example, suggested that the VHA should only concentrate on service-related mental and physical health conditions rather than routine primary care. If treatment of veterans were limited in this fashion, many service-related conditions that experienced VHA providers now identify in primary-care visits would go undetected. Such conditions would be far less likely to be diagnosed by private-sector providers, who often have little knowledge of military or veterans' problems. As Blecker pointed out in his letter of dissent, if Vietnam veterans were dependent on the private sector, PTSD and problems related to Agent Orange, which the VA itself took too long to identify, may never have been recognized and researched at all. (Having learned from its Vietnam experience, the VHA has been quick to identify and act to treat TBI, the signature injury of the wars in Iraq and Afghanistan.)[80]

Also alarming was Veterans' Affairs Committee members' bipartisan embrace of the recommendations by Cosgrove and Schlichting that the VHA abandon its highly successful in-house system of electronic medical recordkeeping (which it is working to improve) and replace it instead with commercial products. Lobbyists for companies that produce these systems[81] have spent millions urging hospitals to purchase their wares— despite the fact that, as a large body of research[82] has documented and as a recent JAMA editorial underscored, they have largely failed to fulfill their promise of creating safer and more efficient healthcare.[83]

"The systems being proposed for purchase at the VHA have been widely disparaged by medical professionals and patient safety advocates for their lack of user friendliness, failure to consider clinical workflow and prioritization of billing information over care," Ross Koppel, an expert in healthcare information technology at the University of Pennsylvania, told me.

During the hearing, no member of Miller's committee expressed concern about the estimated 125,000 veterans whose military discharges— sometimes due to service-related mental health problems—bar them from the VHA. The Commission on Care recommended that some veterans with other than honorable discharge receive tentative eligibility for health-care services.

All in all, it was a disappointing day for vets on Capitol Hill as well as of potential future problems over the next several years.[84]

CHAPTER TWELVE
CONVERSATION WITH A COMMISSIONER

COMMISSION ON CARE MEMBER Phillip Longman, is a senior editor at the *Washington Monthly* and a program director at the New America Foundation. A few days after the Commission on Care released its final report,, I had the opportunity to interview Longman. The following is an edited transcript of our conversation.

<u>Gordon</u>: Can you start by explaining how you came to be on the Commission on Care?

<u>Longman</u>: My main credential was being the author of the book, *Best Care Anywhere: Why VA Care Is Better Than Yours*. In it I described the quality transformation that the VA had undergone in the 1990s and how study after study shows that it still delivers care that, for all its deficiencies, is generally superior to the rest of the U.S. healthcare system. Senator Bernie Sanders knew my work on the VA, and he and I talked several times about it in the context of dealing with the so-called VA "scandal" that broke in 2014. At his request Harry Reid appointed me to the commission. I'd never been on a commission like this before and didn't know what to expect.

<u>Gordon</u>: What most surprised you at the first meeting?

<u>Longman</u>: The commission consisted of six Republican appointees and six Democratic appointees chosen by the leadership of the House and Senate, as well as three appointees named by the White House. The Republican appointees were predictably hostile to the VA, but I was surprised to learn that so were several of the Democratic appointees. One even joined with many of the Republicans in putting forward a plan that aligned perfectly with that of the Koch brothers, while others pushed agendas that also would have effectively privatized the VA.

Gordon: Before we get to that, can you explain a bit about how VA healthcare currently works?

Longman: The VA has long been the only actual example of socialized medicine in the United States. Unlike Medicare and Medicaid, it owns and operates its own hospital clinics, and most of the doctors and other medical professional who work in these facilities are government employees with civil service protections. The VA serves patients with service-related disabilities and/or low incomes, as well as other honorably discharged veterans who meet its eligibility requirements, which change over time.

Gordon: What do you mean by "privatization," and who's for it?

Longman: Over the decades many conservatives have, for ideological reasons, sought to get the VA out of the business of providing healthcare. According to their worldview, the VA must be broken and must be shown to be broken. To them it is axiomatic that government, and by extension socialized medicine, is wasteful and inefficient. Facts showing the VA outperforming the private healthcare system and enjoying overwhelming support from veterans basically contradict their entire worldview and so must be denied.

Most conservatives with this cast of mind propose abolishing the VA altogether and just giving vets vouchers they can use to purchase care from private providers. Senator John McCain is a longtime proponent of this idea. Others, including the Koch brothers and the Astroturf veterans' organization they support, Concerned Veterans for America, would let the VA survive as a vestigial institution but would divert most of its patients to competing networks of private-sector providers.

Many private-sector providers, in turn, love the idea of privatization because it means lot of new patients and lucrative government subsidies flowing their way—particularly if there are few controls over expenditures. This is especially true these days, as American healthcare evolves into a system dominated by giant corporate hospital chains that would very much like to feed off the VA's current patients.

Gordon: Such corporations were well represented on the commission.

Longman: Indeed they were. Three of the commissioners were CEOs of giant healthcare systems, and one was a high-level executive. With one important exception, they pressed hard to get the VA substantially out of the business of being a provider of healthcare. Instead of the VA continuing to compete with them for patients, they wanted the VA to send patients their way. The VA would thus cease to be a provider of healthcare and become a mere payer of healthcare bills submitted by the corporations they represented. At the end of the day, however, all the commissioners affiliated with giant hospital chains overcame their built-in conflict of interest and signed off on a proposal that, while it may incidentally bring some more business their way, does not privatize the VA. I applaud them for that.

Gordon: Are there other reasons people support privatizing the VA?

Longman: Well, some hope, reasonably enough, that allowing VA enrollees to see private-sector doctors will ease the wait times that veterans experience in some facilities for some treatments. They also hope to give vets more choices. Though there are tradeoffs involved, under certain conditions, these are goals worth pursuing.

Improved access and choice were the rationales for the so-called Choice Act that Congress passed with bipartisan support in 2014. That legislation commanded the VA to quickly set up networks of private providers who would be available to treat veterans living more than forty miles from the nearest VA providers or who had to wait more than thirty days for an appointment.

Unfortunately, the program was deeply flawed in design. Because of the very short timelines Congress imposed on its creation, the plan was even worse in execution. The forty miles/thirty days requirement is arbitrary. Most vets who try to use the program have trouble making it work for them because it is administered by private contractors who add an extra layer of bureaucracy. There was no provision for the integration of care between VA and non-VA providers, which creates all sorts of opportunities for medical errors and impacts the quality of care veterans receive.

Gordon: What did the commission propose instead, and why?

Longman: We started with a number of observations, one of the most important being that, in reality, care outside the VA is often very dangerous, as you well know.

Gordon: In fact, preventable medical errors are the third leading cause of death in the United States. I'm also reminded of a story told in Walter Isaacson's biography of Steve Jobs. When Jobs was dying of pancreatic cancer, his wife had to force the myriad specialists who were caring for him to talk to one another. So even a billionaire with the best insurance in the world and more money than God didn't get coordinated care without his wife fighting for it.

Longman: Indeed. One of the things that are unfortunate about how this commission functioned is that we didn't have people come in to testify about how fragmented and dangerous the American healthcare system is. We had people on the commission who were simply unaware, or in denial about, how contact with the U.S. healthcare system kills a quarter of a million Americans a year through a combination of overtreatment, undertreatment, and mistreatment.

Unless one is aware of this reality, one is unable to put the real deficiencies of the VA into context or to think straight about the implications of privatization. When some other commissioners heard about or experienced things that are wrong about the VA, they didn't think to ask the all-important "compared-to-what?" question. They failed to realize, for example, that though wait times are sometimes unacceptably long at the VA, they are on average even longer for most Americans outside the VA, including those who are fully insured.

I and VA supporters on the commission, such as Michael Blecker and David Gorman, and its masterful chairperson, Nancy Schlichting, wanted to preserve the best features of VA care. All VA doctors work off a common electronic medical record, which allows for extensive coordination of care between different specialists, as well as between primary-care and mental health professionals. Unlike fee-for-service doctors in the private sector, VA doctors have no financial incentives tempting them to perform unnecessary surgery or redundant tests. VA clinicians are also typically highly competent when it comes to the physical and mental health issues—particularly those that affect people who have served in the military. These were a key value of VA care that I believe this proposal, if correctly implemented, preserves.

At the same time, however, we recognize that the VA does face capacity constraints in certain areas and that it doesn't always make economic or clinical sense for the VA to produce on its own every single healthcare service it provides. Some veterans live in areas where there are no nearby VA hospitals or clinics. Others may need rare and highly specialized treatment that the VA cannot efficiently provide on its own.

There is nothing really new or different about this. The VA is one of the world's largest purchasers of drugs. It does not follow from this that the VA should run its own pill factories. It does much better for its patients by using its massive purchasing power and clinical expertise to extract value

from private drug companies. Moreover, for years the VA has been contracting for care with providers in the community when that made sense.

Gordon: So what are you proposing that is new?

Longman: We are proposing giving the VA expanded powers and flexibility in contracting for auxiliary capacity. Specifically, we envision the VA
setting up highly integrated networks of very well-credentialed community providers in areas where it lacks the capacity to give timely, high-quality
care to veterans.

Importantly, these community providers will be chosen by the VA itself,
will work off a common VA electronic medical record platform, and will be
accountable for meeting VA clinical performance standards at a set price.
They will work alongside VA employees as part of a coherent, integrated, healthcare delivery system. They will effectively be contract employees
and, as such, will give the VA managers far better ability to adjust capacity
up or down quickly and as needed in different areas.

These networks should increase the choices veterans have in healthcare. But the proposal does not put choice above all other values. Offering
unlimited, unmanaged choice of doctors and treatments would not only
lead to dangerously fragmented care, it would also cost so much that, in
the real world, it would be a political non-starter and thus limit choice.

Two of our commissioners, who both have affiliations with the Koch
brothers, refused to sign the report because they said it did not provide
veterans with sufficient choice. I interpret this to mean that the Kochs feel
more threatened by the specter of socialized medicine succeeding in the
United States than they are by the prospect of the government spending
hundreds of billions of taxpayer dollars to subsidize the services of private-sector healthcare providers. I guess this makes sense if you remember that their plan, though it may inflate government expenditures, essentially amounts to corporate welfare for hospital chains.

Gordon: Some critics, including your fellow commissioner Michael
Blecker, who also refused to sign the report, are concerned that these networks amount to privatization and that their cost will crowd out funding
for traditional VA hospitals and services.

Longman: I understand and respect Michael's concerns, but I believe
strongly that the upsides, for both the vets and VA, are far greater than he
realizes. Most veterans eligible for VA care do not use it or use it only spo-
radically. Three common reasons are that they do not live near a VA facility

or they need a specialty treatment the VA does not offer or they cannot get an appointment as quickly as they would like.

This proposal addresses all those concerns and more. It makes the package of benefits the VA offers superior to what is available today, which means—and this is the key point—more veterans will sign up for VA care. We are not talking about a zero-sum game; we are talking about growing the VA. And expanding the "customer base" for the VA expands the political support for the program and, by extension, for the VA's model of socialized medicine.

Gordon: What would have to happen to realize your vision? The creation of a high-functioning network of outside providers who work in concert, not competition, with those in the VHA is an enormous job. To create an interoperable IT platform, teach outside providers how to do integrated care and talk to one another as well as VA providers, educate them in cultural and military competence—all of this will take a lot of time and money. Congress would, for example, have to allocate more money to the VHA to allow the hiring of staff to engage in the very large job of setting up these networks and would have to make sure that money for care within the VHA is not cannibalized for care outside of it. Is that not correct?

Longman: Yes, setting up these networks will take money, and it will take time. Our mandate was to come up with a twenty-year plan for the VA, and that's how long this plan might take to fully implement. In the report we call on Congress to give VA managers more flexibility in deploying their budget. We also have many other proposals for improving the VA's recruitment and training of managers. This should help prevent poor decision making in how the VA deploys its available resources. If, as I believe, improving the benefit package causes many more eligible veterans to enroll in the VA, then costs will increase commensurately, but there are plans for that as well that the commission recommends be studied.

Gordon: Are you talking about the plan to expand access to VA care to currently ineligible veterans and family members of veterans who have not served in the military?

Longman: I am. The plan is to allow such folks to use their Medicare or private insurance to purchase care within the VA network where sufficient capacity exists or can be made to exist. The VA already has excess capacity in many regions. Moreover, with these new, expanded community networks, we can adjust capacity upwards comparatively easily. Doing so allows the VA to increase its revenues by attracting paying customers, who eventually could include every American. The VA, under this scenario, becomes the means by which the U.S. finally achieves a true public option in healthcare—not just the option to purchase government health insurance, but true socialized medicine.

I could not get a full recommendation out of the commission for this proposal. Veterans' groups such as the American Legion support it. But it ran into opposition from representatives of corporate medicine who concluded, correctly, that it would eventually mean serious competition for their largely monopolistic enterprises.

Nonetheless, I did get the commission to recommend setting up another commission to study the matter. A full description of the plan is also included in the appendix. Just maybe this could turn out to be a big deal in, say, five to ten years, when the American people finally rise up against the abject failures of the rest of the U.S. healthcare system.

Gordon: The VA would also have to do a tremendous amount of outreach to help veterans understand what kind of services the VHA provides and how these services can help them. Right now, as we've seen, many eligible veterans don't enroll in the VHA because of misperceptions about how it works; who is, in fact, eligible for services; and what kind of quality of care it delivers. Congress currently prohibits the VHA from advertising and marketing its services, and most VHA medical centers do not have enough public communications staff to get the message out. This significantly restricts its ability to reach veterans and the public. These communication obstacles need to be addressed if this plan is to work.

Longman: I agree that the VA needs to do a much better job of telling its own story. It would be great if it were allowed to advertise and if it had a more effective communication strategy. Some of the governance changes we make in the report may help with that, particularly the creation of a board of directors that can concentrate on communicating the VA's story to members of Congress and the public at large.

Gordon: This particular recommendation has been very contentious, has it not?

Longman: Some folks have interpreted the language in the report to mean that this board would somehow usurp the power of Congress and the executive branch over the VA—or that, in other words, it constitutes some kind of privatization. But read the substance of the proposal carefully, and you'll see that this is a misreading. The board would include people drawn from the private sector, but this in no way changes the VA's legal status as a government agency accountable to Congress, the White House, and, by extension, the public.

To the disappointment of some conservatives on the commission, we did not recommend that the VA become even a government-sponsored organization like Amtrak or the postal service, let alone a private corporation. With the right members, the board we propose could serve a useful function in advising on strategy and could help insulate VA managers a bit from all the political interference they now get from grandstanding members of Congress. We certainly hope it does. But Congress would still control the VA's budget, and Congress and the White House would together select the members of this board, so, strictly speaking, it would have no independent power.

Gordon: What role do you see veterans' advocacy groups playing in the future of the VA?

Longman: Veterans' groups have an obligation to draw attention to the deficiencies of the VA; that's part of their mission. But it is equally important for them to make sure that the public and its representatives also recognize the excellent services the VA provides and realize that veterans will not stand for privatization of the VA. Disabled American Veterans is playing a particularly valuable role in informing veterans and other stakeholders about the dangers of privatization. They are doing a great job of rebutting the largely false narratives about the VA that are bundled up and promoted by privatizers and often mindlessly recirculated in the press. Since most members of the press, like most members of the public, have no contact with military life or with the VA, effective advocacy is becoming harder and harder to pull off, but also more and more essential.

Gordon: When many non-veterans and people who don't know any veterans read about the debates about the VHA, they may not consider the outcome to have any impact on them whatsoever. I know we both believe that what's at stake in this debate isn't just the quality and cost of healthcare services to veterans, but the future of American healthcare and—even more important—of American government. Can you comment on why you believe the fight for the VHA impacts all of us?

Longman: I believe the VA can become the mechanism by which universal, government-provided healthcare comes to the United States. The

VA model of care, with its emphasis on integration, prevention, and evidence-based, cost-effective care, is also in the forefront of where the rest of the U.S. healthcare needs to go. If we lose the VA, the cause of real healthcare delivery system reform will be set back by at least another generation, with incalculably dire consequences to the health and finances of the American population.

SECTION THREE

THE UNKNOWN STORY

BECAUSE THE NATION'S media have been focused almost exclusively on the problems of the VHA, we barely hear anything about its successes—for example, the scope and importance of its research. How many members of the public know about the VHA's unique partnership with NCIRE, the Veterans Health Research Institute, a nonprofit located at the San Francisco VA Medical Center (SFVAMC), which is the leader in veterans' health research? We also don't hear much of its teaching mission. The VHA has established partnerships with 1,800 educational institutions for health professionals and trains 62,000 medical students and residents each year, as well as 23,000 nursing students and 33,000 health professional students in other fields. About 70 percent of all physicians in the United States have trained at a VHA institution, and it has the largest nursing force in the country. (How all these trainees will be absorbed into a private-sector health system that has trouble accommodating those it must educate now is a question that is rarely addressed in the debate about the VHA's future.)

In this section I provide a glimpse into VHA research and clinical practice, inviting you to explore innovations in the treatment of PTSD and other mental health problems as well as attend conferences on VHA brain research that characterize this massive healthcare system. And please, prepare to breathe deeply and meditate on how integrated care in the VHA connects dots that are too often unlinked in the private sector as patients are asked to be the coordinators of their own care, no matter how complex or arduous the task.

CHAPTER THIRTEEN
HOW VHA RESEARCH SAVES LIVES

ONE OF THE MAIN MISSIONS of the VHA is to conduct research that will improve the health of veterans. In 2015 alone, according to VA Undersecretary for Health David Shulkin, VHA researchers published 9,480 papers in the scientific literature.

In December 2016 the VHA, in partnership with the Prostate Cancer Foundation, embarked on another critical research initiative. The foundation, which has helped fund the research for many major treatments, has donated $50 million to the VHA, making this, Shulkin said, the largest commitment to cancer research the VHA has ever received. CEO and president Dr. Jonathan Simons said the foundation was eager to work with the VHA, not only because it is the largest healthcare system in America, with the most men suffering from prostate cancer in any healthcare system or institution in the United States. The VHA, he said, also provides researchers with a unique opportunity to help solve some of the most vexing riddles about prostate cancer, democratize treatment through its superior telemedicine capacity, and accelerate the pace at which new drugs and treatments are made available to the nation's veterans.

Prostate cancer is the No. 1 cancer diagnosed in the VHA. (For many Vietnam veterans, prostate cancer is the result of exposure to Agent Orange.) The VHA's highly evolved electronic medical record has collected healthcare information on patients that goes back for decades. "This partnership with the VHA has just increased the aperture to get answers to critical questions in prostate cancer research," said Simons.

One of those questions is why African-American men have a 2.4 times greater risk of death from the disease. By having access to these patients and their medical records, Simons explained, researchers can address "the most important cancer disparity we don't understand: why, of 287 different kinds of cancer, even with identical care, prostate cancer is more aggressive and lethal in African-American men. We can finally get to the bottom of what the biological determinants of this are through this partnership with the VHA."

Another thing this new partnership will do is mobilize precision medicine—the use of diagnostic tests to read the DNA code of the cancer to make sure the right treatment is used on the right patient at the right time—to treat prostate cancer. As Simons elaborated, there is no such thing as "prostate cancer." There are over 17 different kinds of prostate cancer. Without reading the DNA code, you risk treating a person with Type 5 prostate cancer using drugs for Type 11.

Working with VHA patients, said Simons, also provides a more representative picture of the actual demographics of American men who suffer from prostate cancer. Without the VHA as a partner, cancer researchers tend to be limited to patients at National Cancer Institute–designated cancer centers or physician group practices. These centers are often located at elite institutions to which many Americans—particularly those in rural areas—lack access. With VHA and its telemedicine system, which is one of the most advanced in the world, says Simons, researchers can work with American cancer patients to create a national network that connects clinical research and the genomics and brings precision oncology to rural areas.

A veteran living in the Black Hills of South Dakota, Shulkin explained, will be able to gain access to any treatments that the partnership develops as easily as someone living in a resource-rich urban area. Because many of the veterans eligible for VHA care are low-income, indigent, or even homeless, and without the VHA might be among the uninsured, both Shulkin and Simons argued that this project will also "democratize" care to populations who would normally be denied such innovative treatments.

Because innovations that start in the VHA do not stay in the VHA, research innovations developed in this partnership will not only benefit VHA patients but have the potential to reduce death and suffering from prostate cancer for men all over the country and the world. This is yet another example of why those trying to gradually dismantle the VHA and privatize its services could jeopardize not only veterans' health but research that will benefit generations to come.[86]

CHAPTER FOURTEEN
EMPOWERING NURSES AND PROVIDING HIGH-QUALITY PATIENT CARE

ON DECEMBER 14, 2016, the VHA amended its medical regulations to "permit full practice authority" to many of the system's nurse-practitioners, a move that immediately drew the ire of the medical community. [87]In so doing, the VHA weighed in on a controversy that has embroiled medicine and nursing for the last fifty years: whether advanced practice registered nurses (APRNs) can operate without direct physician supervision.

Since APRNs appeared on the healthcare stage in 1965 with the enactment of Medicare and Medicaid, physicians have responded with deep ambivalence. Some have embraced them as full members of the healthcare team, whereas others—particularly leaders of organizations like the American Medical Association—have argued that nurses should not function on their own and should always—no matter how much experience they have—work under the direction of doctors. APRNs have consistently argued that they should be allowed to make diagnoses and prescribe treatments without physician supervision.

The Institute of Medicine has recommended APRNs be granted what is known as "full practice authority," and countless studies have documented that APRNs provide safe and effective care at lower costs than physicians.[88] The fight has been waged in various states, twenty-two of which have granted full scope of practice to APRNs. But as a federal employer, the VHA's own internal regulations can supersede state law on nursing practice when there is conflict between state and federal law. The VHA's new ruling, which will establish additional "professional qualifications an individual must possess to be appointed as an APRN within the VA," might actually lead to requirements stricter than those of some states.

This is by no means an arcane, internecine fight. Advanced practice nursing appeared in the 1960s because of the need to expand healthcare access in a country that did not, and still does not, produce enough generalist physicians but overproduces medical specialists. Over the years nurse-practitioners and other APRNs have become increasingly critical in both pediatric and adult primary care, as well as in specialist clinics and acute-care settings where they work on medical teams.

Of the 93,500 registered nurses, licensed practical nurses, and nursing assistants employed by the VHA, more than 5,700 are APRNs hired to work on primary-care teams or in settings with provider shortages. In its deliberations on the future of the VHA, for example, the VA Commission on Care recommended that APRNs be allowed to practice to the full extent of their education, training, and certification, which means without direct physician supervision.

When the VHA's regulation came out, medical leaders expressed their usual reservations about APRN practice. During the sixty-day comment period for the proposed ruling, just the hint of liberating APRN practice unleashed an unprecedented torrent of comments from the American public (including many veterans and their families) and professional organizations. AMA President Andrew Gurman immediately denounced it, saying, "We are disappointed by the VA's decision today to allow most advanced practice nurses within the VA to practice independently of a physician's clinical oversight, regardless of individual state law."[89]

Medical leaders must stop defending an outdated model in which physicians, some of whom may have no training in either leadership or teamwork, dominate the healthcare team. It is time to follow the lead of the VHA and establish a model of care that helps not just veterans but all Americans. And nurses must also fight to maintain, improve, and strengthen the VHA. It has not only taken action to use APRNs to their full scope of practice, it has also given registered nurses (RNs) and licensed vocational nurses (LVNs) as well as other nursing personnel a greater voice in primary care through its Patient Aligned Care Team (PACT) model.[90] The VHA is also one of the only healthcare systems in the country to act to protect nurses from the dangers of lifting heavy patients by installing lift equipment in its hospitals.[91] Just as the VHA has acted to protect nurses, it's time for nurses—and not only those who work at the VHA—to speak up to protect a healthcare system that is focused on protecting RNs and their patients.[92]

CHAPTER FIFTEEN
MAKING PTSD TREATMENT MORE EFFECTIVE

I HAVE SPENT ALMOST THREE YEARS observing caregivers and their patients at the SFVAHCS at Fort Miley. One of the research projects I have observed is an investigation of the impact of killing on veterans who have been in combat and how it influences their response to PTSD treatment. The project's lead investigator is clinical psychologist Shira Maguen, mental health director of the OEF/OIF Integrated Care Clinic and staff psychologist on the Post-Traumatic Stress Disorder Clinical Team (PCT).

Maguen began her research when she worked as an intern and then a postdoctoral fellow at the VHA's National Center for PTSD at the Boston VA Medical Center. She was concerned that a number of her patients who had undergone treatment weren't doing as well as she had hoped. The usual focus of PTSD therapy was on the deprivation or threats the patient had experienced. Was this approach missing something, Maguen wanted to know.

She discovered that the act of killing or witnessing or participating in violence and abuse—particularly of noncombatants—was deeply distressing to some veterans. When she moved to the San Francisco VA Medical Center, Maguen and a team of other mental health clinicians held focus groups with veterans from many different eras. "Many of the people we talked with were suffering tremendously not just because of what was done to them but because of what they did in war."

Veterans who had been in therapy for years told researchers they had never talked about these things and felt terrible guilt, shame, and contamination because of their experiences. "They felt they didn't deserve a family or to have children or to have successful relationships or even be successful in life," said Maguen.

Members of the military were experiencing what is now called moral injury, which happens when people violate moral rules or beliefs. "In war," Maguen elaborates, "people have to make quick decisions." When those wars occur in urban environments like Iraq, this may mean killing a child or civilian who someone thinks may be carrying a gun or who gets caught in a cross fire or explosions.

"Your morality gets tossed out the window," one veteran told researchers. "Same thing with religion, because I think once you start thinking about it—'Boy, I can't do this because this is against everything I've been taught or believed in since I was a young person,'—when you start thinking about the moral issue, you'll be dead. You don't have time to think about those things. You just do it."

Maguen and her colleagues began to measure the impact of killing in three different eras—Vietnam, the Gulf War, and Iraq—and consistently found that killing was associated with PTSD and significant emotional problems that often made it hard for people to function in civilian life. At the SFVAMC the research team held seven focus groups with twenty-six veterans. They used the information and insights they gained to construct a specific measure, called the Killing Cognition Scale (KCS). The KCS captures the various ways that veterans may think about or perceive their past actions. In particular, the KCS tracks the guilt or shame they may experience as well as their ability to forgive themselves or ask for forgiveness from others.

"The KCS helps us get a sense of where veterans are most stuck," says Maguen. "Is their problem guilt? Is it shame or a sense of having been contaminated by their experience? If we understand the distinctions, we can better craft treatments." Guilt, Maguen explains, may lead people to reach out to others to make amends, whereas shame has been linked with reckless risk-taking, social withdrawal, and even decreased empathy for others.

Maguen and her team developed a special treatment, which can supplement others, to deal with killing and moral injury. In a randomized control trial jointly funded by the University of California at San Francisco (UCSF) and the VHA, one group of veterans received six to eight weeks of a specially designed treatment called The Impact of Killing (IOK). The control group, some of whom were already in PTSD treatment, had to wait for six weeks to receive the newer therapeutic intervention. They were allowed to continue their groups or individual therapy but not engage in prolonged exposure therapy or cognitive processing therapy, which are the gold standard treatments for PTSD.

Those patients who received IOK therapy began by filling out the KCS so therapists could gain a nuanced understanding of their symptoms. Then, in individual therapy sessions, they learned about the physiological responses to killing and how they are connected to emotions and thoughts. Therapists then explored their feelings of guilt, shame, or contamination. The most important sessions of all, Maguen notes, are those that consider self-forgiveness. This process of asking for forgiveness and self-forgiveness, Maguen says, is not designed to deny or condone problematic actions but rather to help veterans get a reprieve after years of self-punishment, which may involve divorces, estrangement from children, lost jobs, alcohol and drug abuse, and long stints of homelessness.

Veterans are asked to write a forgiveness letter. Some write letters to the person they killed, to a village they may have harmed, or even to their younger self. At the end of the treatment, they read their forgiveness letter to their therapist. Like those who have gone through twelve-step programs, this therapy also includes some form of making amends.

Maguen explains: "The amends are focused on, 'Okay, you are starting the process of self-forgiveness, so what are you going to do to make an action plan moving forward? How are you going to reach out to anyone your behavior may have hurt? How are you going to talk to your spouse? What about kids who may be estranged? Is there community service you might choose to perform?' Part of the amends process could also involve reconnecting to a religious or spiritual community." After the process of amends, the patient and the therapist create a forgiveness and amends plan for the future, thus assuring that the therapeutic experience is not only present but sustainable over the long term.

After this randomized control trial, Maguen and her colleagues found that those who participated in the treatment had reduced mental health and PTSD symptoms. Depression and anxiety symptoms were also reduced. Veterans were able to be more intimate with a partner, ruminated less on bad experiences, and engaged in more community events. As they forgave themselves, they were able to be more compassionate and accepting of others. The researchers are publishing a paper on this innovative therapy and hope to roll it out at multiple VHA facilities across the country.

In the debate about VHA privatization, there has been a great deal of discussion of shifting more mental health services to the private sector. One must ask whether the kind of research Maguen and others are doing would be possible if veterans were seen by private-sector professionals who only had a scattering of former service members in their practices and little experience with the nuances of military-related PTSD. Or is this kind of work dependent on the VHA's large, national community of clinicians and researchers who deliver healthcare to a very particular population of patients?

When I asked Maguen these questions, she said: "This work would not be possible in the private sector because the majority of psychologists, psychiatrists, social workers, psychiatric NPs, whomever, would probably not specialize in a veteran population. Even those who treat PTSD might have some veterans scattered among their patients. This would not provide the kind of volume that leads to the kind of questioning that goes on in an institution, where everyone treated is a veteran and has shared a certain set or at least subset of experiences." Hopefully, Congress will heed this insight as it considers the fate of the VHA.[93]

CHAPTER SIXTEEN
THE BRAIN AT WAR

EACH YEAR NCIRE PUTS on a research conference entitled "The Brain at War," which spotlights leading researchers who, in partnership with UCSF, produce fascinating insights and treatments to deal with health-care issues that affect veterans. The advances produced by this research, as well as all other VHA research, have ripple effects far beyond the veteran population.

In October 2015 the theme of the conference was "Mending Minds and Wounds: Returning Health to Those Returning Home."[94] Although many of us might think that the biggest problem that bring veterans to the VHA is TBI or PTSD, it is, in fact, tinnitus—that ringing of the ears that comes with hearing loss in aging. The veteran population is far older than those treated in other healthcare systems. The average veteran is sixty-two, and many are much older. So tinnitus would be a big problem for them even if they hadn't served in the military. My husband, who is not a veteran, had to visit a hearing specialist to get help with his ear ringing. I notice mine late at night, when I am falling asleep.

Veterans have even more problems with hearing loss because the conditions of their work subject them to the kind of loud, percussive noises that damage the ear. As researcher Steven W. Cheung, MD, staff physician on the Surgical Service at SFVAHCS and professor of otolaryngology at UCSF, pointed out in his presentation, "Advances in Tinnitus Imaging and Treatment," there is no part of the military where service members can avoid the kind of loud noises that produce tinnitus. The constant hum on ships impacts the ears of sailors; the whirr of engines does damage to airmen and -women; and those in the marines and army are subjected to a constant barrage of artillery fire and explosives, even in training. I met one patient at the VHA who had hearing loss and tinnitus because he served in Arlington National Cemetery, where he shot off guns all day as part of the standard salute at military funerals. This was during the Vietnam era, and he and his fellow soldiers wore no protective hearing gear.

For most people tinnitus is a minor annoyance. For 3 percent of people who have it, it's problematic, and for 0.5 percent, it severely disrupts normal life. As Cheung described it, for those sufferers, tinnitus is a form of chronic auditory pain. Although a lot of people think of tinnitus as an ear problem, Cheung explained that it's a problem that involves the whole brain. To deal with that, researchers at UCSF, the VHA, and NCIRE have utilized research they have conducted on people whose brains have been impacted by Parkinson's disease. They have discovered that patients undergoing deep brain stimulation (DBS) had a dramatic reduction in severity of symptoms (loudness) from their tinnitus.

In the course of his talk, Cheung showed an amazing video of a veteran who had been treated with DBS for the motor problems brought on by Parkinson's disease. In the first segment of the short video, the veteran could barely get up from his chair and make it across a room. In the second, after DBS, he practically bounded out of his seat and launched himself almost missile-like across the space in front of him. It was quite a sight. Inspired by what can be achieved for patients with Parkinson's disease, Cheung and his colleagues hope DBS will bring meaningful relief for those who suffer from tinnitus.

This complex treatment is promising for people whose lives are made an auditory nightmare by tinnitus, which again includes far more patients than those in the veteran population. I couldn't help thinking, for example, about what the ears of all those young people hanging around nifty bars or restaurants in San Francisco would be like after age 45, when hearing loss normally begins. Or how about those poor bartenders and wait staff subjected to that percussive force day in and day out? Maybe some of them will benefit from VHA research.

Another session of the conference dealt with "Innovative Approaches to Mental Health." Veterans suffer from a variety of complex problems, sometimes brought on by military service, sometimes exacerbated by it. These include PTSD and insomnia, which again, are not problems exclusive to the veteran population. In one presentation Thomas C. Neylan, MD, professor of psychiatry at UCSF and director of the Stress and Health Research Program at SFVAHCS, described a study that was funded by the DOD and conducted by SFVAHCS. The study compared two different sleep medications, zolpidem (Ambien) and almorexant. The study focused on the cognitive side effects of these drugs. Pharma-funded studies comparing one drug's effectiveness, or even side effects, against another's are rare. Few pharmaceutical companies are interested in potentially demonstrating that one of their medications is not as good as one produced by another company.

In his presentation Neylan reported that the study showed that almorexant had fewer cognitive side effects than zolpidem. Although the company that developed almorexant, Actelion, has stopped its work on the medication, a cousin of this drug, suvorexant, has been approved by the FDA, and others in this class are being developed.

As Neylan explained to me, "The cognitive side effects of sleeping medication result in accidents and injuries. People get up in the middle of the night to use the bathroom or are awakened in the middle of the night unexpectedly. The worry is that if you are awakened under the influence of a sleeping medication, you are at higher risks of injuries and accidents and making mistakes because of the cognitive side effects of sleeping pills. So a new sleeping medication that has fewer cognitive side effects would be important to a very large population."

As someone who has taken zolpidem (who hasn't?) for occasional sleep problems, I can certainly attest to the relevance of a study to millions of people like me who have never seen a battlefield or been trained to perform on one.

Another presentation shifted the focus to the social and emotional aspects of veterans' problems. In her presentation on dealing with chronic pain, Karen Seal, MD, PhD, director of the Integrated Pain Team at SFVAHCS and professor of medicine and psychiatry at UCSF, discussed a different approach—an integrative rather than biomedical approach to the kind of chronic pain that many veterans experience. Rather than searching for a silver bullet medication—say, opioids—to treat pain, her work looks at how those who treat chronic pain can integrate other kinds of treatments, for example, yoga, that are proven to help with pain while avoiding the downside of opioid use and abuse. At SFVAHCS, chronic pain groups now emphasize restoration of function and refer patients for acupuncture, chiropraxis, and relaxation techniques, among other things. Over 100 million Americans suffer from chronic pain. Chronic pain costs the nation about $600 million a year. The success of such an approach in the veteran population could clearly help those treated outside the VHA system as well.

Over several years the VHA has received little praise for the excellent care it provides the nation's veterans. Many Republicans in Congress, pushed and prodded by the Koch brothers–financed CV A, are trying to promote partial or even complete privatization of the VHA.[95] Members of the public, swayed by a barrage of all too often highly exaggerated accounts of VHA failings (failings, for example, by one hospital that are used to tarnish an entire system) may support these proposals. What they ignore are the many accomplishments of the nation's largest integrated healthcare system. That's why conferences like "The Brain at War" are so important. They remind us of these accomplishments and the significant research mandate the VHA fulfills. It is hard to imagine how this research would be funded and conducted in the private healthcare system. But it is easy to imagine how veterans and many others would suffer without it.

CHAPTER SEVENTEEN
SUICIDE BY GUN

IN AMERICA'S RANCOROUS DEBATE about gun control, the focus tends to be on homicides, particularly mass shootings. In reality, far more lives are lost every day through firearm-assisted suicide. There are nearly twice as many suicides by gun annually as there are murders involving guns. With these stats, and a particular at-risk population in mind, the San Francisco VA Healthcare System (VAHCS) and the American Foundation for Suicide Prevention's Greater San Francisco Bay Area Chapter held a conference in San Francisco on March 4, 2016, aimed at reducing suicides among veterans by getting more of them to safely store their firearms and "other lethal means."

Presenters and participants at the "Counseling Veterans at Risk for Suicide: Safe Storage of Firearms and Other Lethal Means" conference included former military personnel who had contemplated or even attempted suicide, the parents of a young soldier who succeeded, mental healthcare professionals, suicide prevention researchers, and three firearms dealers. All agreed that one way to reduce the number of veterans killing themselves (now estimated at twenty a day nationally) is to promote safe storage, an approach backed by public health researchers and mental health clinicians.

The March 4 conference was not just for the already convinced, however. It was designed to find common ground with those resistant (for political or emotional reasons) to any measures perceived as reducing rather than increasing personal safety and security. As Russell Lemle, PhD, psychology director at the San Francisco SFVAHCS and one of the conference organizers, acknowledged, "If we are going to forge effective approaches in the broader veteran community, we need the voices of gun advocates, veterans, and their families."

In her introductory speech, Christine Moutier, MD, chief medical officer for the American Foundation for Suicide Prevention, explained that suicides are now the tenth leading cause of death in the United States, with firearms the means of choice in half of successful attempts. Psychologists Caitlin Thompson, the national leader in suicide prevention for the VHA, and Megan McCarthy, the lethal means safety coordinator at the SFVHCS, explained that although the suicide rate for older veterans is the same as that of their counterparts in the general population, the rate for younger veterans from the wars in Iraq and Afghanistan is higher. Seventy percent of all the veterans who succeed in taking their own lives do so with firearms.

Jean and Howard Somers, mother and father of one of these veterans, told the story of their son, Daniel Somers, a sergeant in the California Army National Guard. In 2013, after years of coping with the aftermath of numerous TBIs and PTSD acquired during multiple combat missions in Iraq, he wrote his parents and wife that he was, "Too trapped in a war to be at peace, too damaged to be at war . . . My body has become nothing but a cage, a source of pain and constant problems." He took his firearm and ended his life.[96]

Jason Zimmerman, a former army medic who has PSTD and is now a peer specialist at the James H. Quillen VA Medical Center in Mountain Home, Tennessee, explored one of the central dilemmas the conference addressed. For many veterans, gun ownership is part of their culture. "In the military service," Zimmerman explained, "we learned that our weapons are our friends."

Once out of the service, Zimmerman continued, veterans may be reluctant to go into counseling or report a mental health problem or suicidal thoughts because they erroneously believe their weapons will be taken away from them. They and their families will then be unprotected from threatening strangers, which many report to be the primary reason they own firearms.

To reduce the threat of suicide in a population committed to gun ownership, therefore, is a challenge. One that can be addressed, conference participants argued, by promoting the safe storage of weapons. Catherine Barber, director of the Means Matter project at the Harvard School of Public Health's Injury Control Research Center, explained that many members of the public believe that people who try to kill themselves will find a way to succeed. Scientific evidence, she explained, dispels this myth: Suicide is usually an impulsive act, and only 10 percent of those who attempt to kill themselves will go on to later die by suicide.

Over and over again, Barber outlined the facts: reducing access to the most lethal means reduces the overall suicide rate. In Sri Lanka, for example, banning the pesticides that were most toxic to humans (the method of choice for a rural population) reduced the overall suicide rate in that country by 50 percent. In England and Wales, when nontoxic gas replaced toxic gas in ovens, suicide rates dropped by 30 percent. In 2006, when the Israel Defense Forces required service members to store their weapons on base when they went on weekend leave, the suicide rate dropped by 40 percent.

For good reason then, suicide prevention advocates and researchers want veterans in crisis to leave their guns with friends or store them at shooting ranges or in safes in their own homes. To encourage veterans to do this, of course, involves asking them the right questions in the right way and at the right time. To make sure this happens, the VHA has funded McCarthy and her colleagues at the SFVAHCS, in collaboration with the Harvard School of Public Health Means Matter project, to develop a pilot project to train mental health providers in lethal means safety counseling. Even seasoned mental health professionals, McCarthy told the audience, need to understand that directly telling a veteran he or she shouldn't have access to a firearm during a crisis will not work as well as guiding the veteran to think about how to keep himself safe when things look unremittingly bleak. The training has been piloted in San Francisco as well as at the VHA in Northern California and four VHA facilities in Pennsylvania and will be disseminated in other VHAs this year.

As is typical with public–private partnerships in the VHA, all the information, research, treatments, and trainings the VHA develop are available to private-sector researchers and practitioners. This is why researchers like Catherine Barber and Christine Moutier, among others, told me they were so impressed with the VHA. "I don't understand the image the media is painting of the VHA," Barber told me candidly. "It bears no relationship to what I see happening and what I experience when working with VHA providers and researchers."

It's a shame that so few members of the media who had been invited attended the conference. The mainstream media seem only interested in reporting negative stories about the largest and only integrated publicly funded healthcare system in the United States. As a result, there have been few media reports on the many research studies documenting the high quality of VHA care for those who have access to it. For example, a recent national study of suicides that occurred between 2000 and 2010 documented that veterans who used VHA services had reduced rates of suicides, whereas veterans not utilizing the VHA had increased rates.[97] Moreover, veterans who seek mental health treatment at the VHA[98] receive care that is far superior to the services offered in the private sector.[99] Veterans who don't know the facts, however, may not seek treatment from the one healthcare system that—when properly funded by Congress—is best equipped to help them.[100]

CHAPTER EIGHTEEN
MINDFULNESS AT FORT MILEY

IT IS TUESDAY AFTERNOON at three o'clock, and four unlikely students of mindfulness meditation are relearning how to breathe. Instruction in being more mindful is everywhere these days, particularly in the Bay Area, so I could have been sitting through a similar training in Berkeley with a group of sixty-something women with crinkling faces, flowing gray hair, and a history of New-Age enthusiasms. Or I could have been on Valencia Street in San Francisco, epicenter of that city's techie takeover, where whiz kids in their twenties and thirties are coping with long hours in Silicon Valley at a studio with a website called stressreductionatwork. com.

The twelve-week mindfulness training I am attending takes place in a distinctly different setting, however. It's held in a corner conference room in Building Number 8, the Behavioral Health Building, at the San Francisco VAHCS at Fort Miley and led by clinical psychologist Susanna Fryer and psychology intern Ian Ramsey. The group of veterans in their fifties and sixties who've come to Fort Miley are not here only for an intellectual or spiritual exercise. For some of these men, becoming better able to control their thoughts and anxieties through mindfulness is literally a matter of life or death.

Dressed in spanking fresh jeans and a starched white shirt, Harvey holds himself steel-rod straight. He speaks deliberately, each word clipped, sharpened as if surrounded by barbed wire and warning signs advising people to keep their distance. His cross to bear is obsessive–compulsive disorder, along with depression and ten years of being homeless.

Ronald, an African-American veteran, is almost his opposite, supple, fluid, and easy with jokes. Yet he has experienced similar struggles with homelessness, poverty, drugs, and divorce.

James has suffered for years from a panic disorder. He will find himself in a supermarket or on a bus suddenly overwhelmed with anxiety. He feels he has to get out or he will, quite literally, die. There have been times when he has run out of the room screaming in fear. These panic attacks have been with him since he was twenty-two, when he was raped during a hazing ritual on a ship when he was in the navy. He is now in his late fifties. For over thirty years, he has self-medicated with drugs and alcohol. He lost job after job and lived on the streets.

Finally, there is Jose, a Vietnam vet who has PTSD, is plagued by nightmares, and has trouble sleeping. A divorce tipped him over the edge, and after twenty years managing without treatment, he went into a spiral of alcohol abuse that led to homelessness before he finally came to the VHA for help.

All of these men struggle just to get from day to day. When they talk about intrusive thoughts, it's not about the boss who wants them to work morning, noon, and night or what diet they should choose, paleo or gluten-free. The things that are a struggle for me—standing in line at the supermarket or a ten-minute wait on hold with some clerk at my doctor's office, are not just some of life's minor, albeit often infuriating, frustrations. For these men they are triggers that can send them into a tailspin from which it can take years to recover.

When they talk about difficult relationships, "negative people," as Ronald describes them, they are talking about a whole lot of people who have ripped them off (or who maybe they have ripped off) who have knives, guns, needles, and bottles into which they can disappear for months at a time.

In many articles on the VHA, reporters talk about veterans' frustration with wait times. Those of us who do not have these problems, naturally assume, "Oh, these guys were frustrated because they had to wait weeks or months to get help." And maybe that was the case. But I have learned that, to someone with PTSD, a TBI, or panic disorder—or all three, an intolerable wait can be fifteen minutes. It could be standing in line for five minutes, not waiting for an appointment for five months.

Susanna Fryer, who facilitates mindfulness-based stress management groups at the SFVAHCS, explains that her work is largely based on pioneering program development by mindfulness advocates including Jon Kabat-Zinn, Zindel Segal, and others. The Fort Miley programs (available at many VHAs across the country), which combine mindfulness and cognitive behavior therapy principles, usually have eight to ten veterans per group. Unlike private-sector programs run on a fee-for-service basis, the VHA's will continue even if some vets drop out. Not all veterans who are referred to the mindfulness program have mental illnesses, Fryer adds. Some with heart disease, for example, or dealing with cancer treatment, may be referred to lower their stress levels. Others may be in chronic pain.

Whatever reason the veterans have for coming, mindfulness training is part of an integrated approach that includes other therapies. The men in the room may have done cognitive behavioral therapy for psychosis, PTSD, depression, or anxiety. They have done group therapy or had an inpatient hospitalization. Some are also taking psychiatric medications.

The mindfulness stress management group, Fryer explains, can complement other treatments. In sessions that build upon one another, veterans learn, and begin to practice, skills that can be used in their daily lives to help them stay connected socially, manage stress, and create healthy habits that will help them be less reactive in the ways that can lead to problems at home or at work.

The idea here is to begin accepting the thoughts that intrude as you concentrate on breathing in, breathing out, eating a raisin, or learning not to focus on people whom you can hear talking through the open window. The goal is to help patients learn to distinguish between the points of the triangle that Fryer always draws on the conference room's whiteboard before she begins each session. At the apex of the triangle is the word "thoughts." At the base, the line connecting to the left edge leads to a point where she writes the word "feelings" Across the bottom another line links "feelings" to "behavior." Thoughts produce feelings—anxiety, depression, anger—which in turn lead to behaviors that can be destructive and danger-ous to ourselves and others. Mindfulness techniques that teach people to tune in to their present-moment experiences can help people understand that a thought is not reality and feelings don't have to lead to destructive behavior.

For example, in one of the sessions I attend, she asks the men to imag-ine a situation. "You're walking down the street, and someone cuts you off. What might be the thought that runs through your head?"

"Get out of my space," Ronald says. "What a jerk, I should have brought my gun."

"I should tell him off," Harvey volunteers.

"This person doesn't know you," Ian Ramsey suggests.

"Let's workshop each of these thoughts," Fryer proposes. "What are you feeling when you think, 'Get out of my space'?"

"Agitated, angry. I feel nervous when people get in my space—nau-seous, even," Ronald explains.

"Retaliation," Harvey adds.

"Like you're entitled?" Fryer probes, "This is my space."

The men continue to explore, discussing the rudeness they see every-where today in San Francisco, the sense that they constantly need to be on the defensive and even to act to defend themselves. As they go deeper, they recognize and discuss the stress response, the lingering impact it has on their mind and body. After further discussion Fryer asks them to consid-er the cycle: something happens, a thought emerges and then influences what they feel and do. "With mindful awareness of your thoughts," she reminds them, "you have other choices."

"That's what I like about this class," James says. "I've got choices I never had before. I get to think about things, not just react. I was at the pharmacy and had to wait in line and got all agitated. Now I can breathe through it instead of reacting like I used to, storming off, furious."

Fryer introduces the acronym HALT to discuss common stress triggers and what happens when people are Hungry, Angry, Lonely, or Tired and how to apply the mindfulness skills from the group to cope when you're in an agitated state. The men nod in agreement. Jose says that sometimes he now says a prayer to relax himself. Harvey goes back to the visualization they have all learned where you let negative thoughts, like leaves, float downstream, until they are far, far away.

Fryer affirms their progress, explaining how the quick, judging brain works to send us off on a negative spiral, making assumptions about the person who cut us off, didn't respond to our needs, or wasn't quick enough to get us our meds. "At the end of the day, we don't even know if people meant what we think they meant."

"Or even if they did, is our response worth it?" Ramsey says.

The group continues discussing how to work with thoughts in a mindful space to cultivate nonjudgmental awareness. "'This being human is a guest house. Every morning a new arrival. A joy, a depression, a meanness, some momentary awareness comes as an unexpected visitor. Welcome and entertain them all. Even if they are a crowd of sorrows,'" Fryer reads from a poem by Rumi called the "The Guest House," commonly recited in mindfulness circles.

Ronald returns to the struggle of waiting on lines, for example, at the checkout counter of the supermarket. After eight sessions of mindfulness work, not only in these weekly hourlong sessions but through homework and practicing mindfulness techniques, he explains that he is trying to get patient with his impatience. He is making strides.

"That's why we call it practice," Ramsey says. "That's why we are here."

EPILOGUE

TRUMP AND THE VHA

PRIOR TO NOVEMBER 8, 2016, Donald Trump repeatedly promised to respect and care for veterans. Yet on the campaign trail, Trump, who never served in the military, called Senator John McCain, who was a navy pilot during the Vietnam War, a "loser" because McCain was shot down in combat and captured. Then Trump attacked a Gold Star military family and dissed mentally ill veterans for being weak.[101] On another occasion he helped raise money for veterans in need but delayed writing a check for his own promised $1-million donation to relevant charities. (That pledge was redeemed only after reporters covering the Trump campaign discovered his foot-dragging and published embarrassing stories about it.)[102]

As both a contender for the White House and president, Trump has surrounded himself with critics, rather than defenders, of the VA. On the campaign trail, he promised to make Congressman Jeff Miller, the House Veterans' Affairs Committee chair, his new secretary of veterans' affairs. Later, Pete Hegseth, former CEO of CVA and a FOX News commentator, was reportedly in the running for the job. In *Apprentice*-like fashion, Trump also interviewed Toby Cosgrove for the job. Fortunately, for the second time in three years, Cosgrove withdrew his name as a candidate for the post.

Trump refused to personally meet with any members of real VSOs. He did, however, hold a widely publicized discussion at his Mar-a-Lago estate with high-ranking executives of hospital systems that would benefit financially from privatization of the VHA. These top administrators included Cosgrove as well as Paul Rothman, CEO of Johns Hopkins Medicine; David Torchiana, CEO of Partners HealthCare in Massachusetts; and John H. Noseworthy, president of the Mayo Clinic. At this meeting Trump asked these executives—who have no experience of providing VHA-style integrated healthcare—to form an advisory committee that will help him in reshaping the agency.[103]

Darin Selnick, executive director of the CVA's Fixing Veterans Health Care taskforce, was named a Trump administration transition advisor. At a post-election meeting of the American Association of Medical Colleges in Seattle, Selnick openly promoted the VA privatization agenda. He argued for putting vets into a tax-supported, private insurance program like TRICARE, which covers active-duty military personnel and their families.

Excluded from Trump's VA transition team were any representatives of the DAV, VFW, or Vietnam Veterans of America, which have hundreds of thousands of members and opposed privatization. When these and other advocacy groups urged the president-elect to retain incumbent Veterans Affairs Secretary Robert McDonald, Trump advisor Newt Gingrich lashed out at them in an interview with the *Washington Post.*

"The Veterans Administration is a total disgrace, and it's embarrassing that the senior veterans' organizations endorsed the current veterans' secretary because he has failed totally to clean it up," Gingrich said. The former Republican House speaker urged Trump to wage "straight-out war" on the whole federal bureaucracy, starting with the VA, which Gingrich singled out for being the "archetype of disaster." In his anti-VA rant, Gingrich questioned why "people who we know broke the rules and killed veterans" should "stay in their jobs."[104]

Gingrich's proposed war on the VHA is not popular among veterans or with their advocacy organizations. Thus, groups like the CVA try to mask their ultimate objectives and insist they are not trying to privatize the VHA. In a report entitled "Fixing Veterans Health Care," the CVA claimed, for example, that it just wants to give veterans "the same degree of choice available to other Americans." In a *New York Times* debate with Phillip Longman, CVA's Arvik Roy similarly argued that "Veterans Should Enjoy the Same Health Care Options as All Americans."[105]

The CVA conveniently ignores the fact that many Americans continue to have no healthcare choices at all because they are uninsured. Even those with insurance have significant coverage limitations. Before Trump's inauguration, and with his unstinting support, the current Republican leadership on Capitol Hill launched an effort to end the federally subsidized, private health insurance coverage that millions of Americans have obtained through the Affordable Care Act. They are also attacking Medicare and Medicaid, no matter how cost-effective, accessible, or popular these programs may be. How much choice will millions of Americans have if attacks on Obamacare, Medicare, and Medicaid succeed?

The CVA also argues that its Choice proposals, as well as those of legislators discussed in earlier chapters, do not constitute privatization. In December 2016 *Washington Post* fact checker Michelle Ye Hee Lee concurred when she awarded Senator Jon Tester (D—Mont.) and Congressman Mark Takano (D—Calif.) three Pinocchios for arguing against CVA-style privatization. The CVA, she wrote, "has not proposed a wholesale transfer of VHA's services over to the private sector—which is what 'privatization' usually describes."[106]

Lee's interpretation flies in the face of volumes of academic and policy research on the privatization movement that went mainstream in the 1980s, notably in the United States and Britain. As Princeton University Professor Paul Starr correctly noted in an essay thirty years ago, privatization is "any shift of activities or functions from the state to the private sector; any shift of production of goods and services from public to private."[107] This process includes (and often begins with) what Starr calls "privatization by attrition"—the incremental transfer of service provision responsibility to private vendors, with an accompanying underfunding of the government agency or department whose scope of activity is curtailed. As Starr and other critics point out, the privatization movement decreases accountability and oversight of services currently delivered by the private sector.

According to Starr, outsourcing advocates invariably try to erode public support for the idea that government can ever play a positive role in meeting social needs. The privatization movement is also closely linked to attacks on public-sector employees and the unions that represent them. Government workers are accused of being incompetent, lazy, uncaring, or even corrupt—a blanket characterization designed to justify denying them any workplace rights. Most privatizers believe that public employees should become what is known as "employees at will." As such, they could be summarily dismissed without cause. They would be allowed no opportunity to rebut allegations made against them in any kind of fair hearing. This would discourage many from speaking up to protect their patients, if ever at risk, or blowing the whistle on ineffective, dangerous, or even corrupt management practices because of fear of employer retaliation.

When it comes to the VHA, would-be privatizers employ the same standard tactics. Although some high-level VHA employees may be guilty of incompetence, mismanagement, or gaming the system in an improper manner, this is certainly not true of the vast majority. Yet those who favor dismantling the VHA have launched an attack on the workplace rights of federal employees. In introducing a bill to make it easier to fire VA employees, Jeff Miller, for example, argued that, "The biggest obstacle standing in the way of VA reform is the department's pervasive lack of accountability among employees at all levels. Until this problem is fixed once and for all, long-term efforts to reform VA are doomed to fail. . . . Union bosses and defenders of the broken status quo will oppose this bill, and that is exactly why it must become law."[108]

This assault is part of a larger, factually challenged narrative, echoed in Gingrich's comments and those made by Donald Trump on the campaign trail and in post- election pronouncements—namely, that the VHA is broken, unaccountable, and repairable only through market-based reforms. As this argument is advanced, any shortcomings in private-sector healthcare delivery that might rival or exceed any in the VHA get Photoshopped out of the picture.

This is why, Harvey Feigenbaum, Jeffrey Henig, and Chris Hamnett persuasively argue, "Treating privatization as one among many politically neutral policy options to be considered by public officials...obscures the underlying political dimension that has given the privatization movement much of its vigor and controversy."[109] In reality what seems almost politically neutral is in fact a radical restructuring scheme that would shift much current funding to private-sector providers. Because each dollar spent in the private sector would come out of the VHA's budget, it would mean less money for the nation's only fully integrated healthcare system. Plus, each veteran who seeks care in the private sector would mean fewer patients in the VHA, which would, in turn, deprive VHA professionals of their ability to maintain a high level of clinical and research expertise by treating the specific service-related problems presented by a large patient population.

As more veterans seek private-sector care that might be of lower quality yet far more expensive than that delivered in the VHA, retaining existing staff and recruiting new employees would be adversely affected. Relentless media attacks and the failure to offer private-sector salaries have already increased the annual loss rate of VHA employees from 7.3 to 8.2 percent. If this continues, even more may leave the agency.

This would inevitably lead to facility closures and staff layoffs. Many of these layoffs would affect the 115,000 VA employees who are themselves veterans. The majority of these veterans, most of whom have service-connected disabilities, work as clerks, housekeepers, emergency room security or transport workers, groundskeepers, VA police, and food-service workers, among others. These workers would find it very difficult to find any employment elsewhere, much less work that provides a living wage and benefits. Privatizers who say they are committed to veterans fail to acknowledge the fact that their proposals jeopardize the careers of veterans with service-connected disabilities who are committed to serving other veterans.

Veterans would also suffer because the VHA shields its patients from unnecessary tests and treatments common in for-profit healthcare chains as well as in hospitals that are sometimes "not-for-profit" in name only. There, doctors and hospitals operating on a fee-for-service basis often have financial incentives to overtreat patients, sometimes urging on them toxic, even futile, medications and procedures that may worsen rather than improve an individual's health.

Patients and their families with private insurance end up buried in bureaucratic paperwork, including ever-increasing bills for co-payments, deductibles, and premium payments. The CVA approach would similarly shift costs to veterans through out-of-pocket payments and mechanisms like interest-bearing health savings accounts. If adopted by Congress, the CVA's plan could also limit eligibility for care in the private sector—or in what remains of the VHA—to veterans who have service-related conditions or were in combat. This radical change would be most harmful to the many low-income and indigent veterans who currently qualify for VA health coverage.

Similarly, it could deny care to 39-year-old veteran Demond Wilson, who spent eighteen years in the marines—none in combat—and who was completely paralyzed after a car accident that occurred after he left the service. After being discharged from Kaiser because his benefits ran out, Wilson turned to the VHA. Today, the VHA provides his sister with a stipend for some of his care. Thanks to a variety of physical and psychological rehabilitation programs, he has recovered limited mobility in his hands, participated in sports, reconnected with his family, and is on his way to returning to work. Without the VHA, he says, he would be left to the mercy of poorly resourced county services, probably destitute, homeless, and too dejected to be a father to his four children or capable of returning to productive work.

A CONTINUED CALL TO ACTION

As I finished writing this book, Donald Trump finally announced his pick for secretary of the Department of Veterans Affairs. Although he rejected the pleas of VSOs who wanted Robert McDonald to continue in the position, he did choose David J. Shulkin, who has served under McDonald as undersecretary for health at the VA. Shulkin actually supports the mission of the agency he will lead and has the qualifications and experience to do the job effectively. This represents a lobbying victory for VSOs and their allies.

Shulkin is not a veteran, but he has worked with McDonald to remedy vexing system problems. His published writings, public testimony, and policy proposals have demonstrated his grasp of the existing system's considerable strengths. In March 2016, in the *New England Journal of Medicine*, Shulkin reminded readers that the VA outperforms private industry in "lower risk-adjusted mortality rates, better patient-safety statistics, and better performance on a number of other accepted process measures."[110] He does not oppose veterans getting care in the private sector when needed but wants the VHA to coordinate and integrate care within the VHA system.

Shulkin has also been outspoken in explaining how the VHA saves lives through its unfairly maligned Veterans Crisis Line.[111] Under Shulkin and McDonald, the VA added a second Veterans Crisis Line in Atlanta to the one operating in rural Canandaigua, New York. Shulkin understands that locating a crisis line in a major urban area will facilitate recruitment of more staff to perform a very arduous job. These dedicated staff listen to veterans in crisis—many of them at risk of suicide or posing a danger to their families, friends, and community members—hour after hour, day after day.

Most important, Shulkin has consistently countered conservative talking points that government can do no right and the private sector no wrong. After more than twenty-five years practicing as both a physician and hospital executive in the private sector, Shulkin has cogently outlined the facts in speeches, interviews, and articles like the one that appeared in *The Federal Practitioner*. The VHA is the only system, he wrote, that has developed expertise in the specific, service-related health problems of its veteran patients. Unlike private-sector providers who pay lip service to the concept of team-based, patient-centered care, the VHA practices what it preaches. Plus, unlike the private sector, the VHA pays attention to issues of poverty and homelessness, integrates mental health into primary care, and even supports family members or friends who are caring for veterans. And in an astonishing prediction for a future Trump cabinet member, Shulkin argued that the VA "can lead the way in advancing the nation's health care. This is the appropriate role for government: Do what the private sector cannot or will not do, given the nature of its enterprise."[112]

If Shulkin is allowed to utilize his knowledge and experience—and apply his moral convictions—to his new role, then all veterans and their allies will be better off. Unfortunately, he will be under much pressure from Congress and the White House to adopt bad policies. Despite the VHA's recent progress on reducing wait times, Trump argued during his press conference announcing Shulkin's nomination that veterans are treated "very unfairly" and that they have to wait "fifteen, sixteen, seventeen days for an appointment." (The average wait in the private sector is nineteen days.) Trump even claimed that some veterans whose appointments were delayed and who had early-stage cancers became terminally ill in just a couple of weeks. The president-elect also announced that he had assembled a brain trust of private-sector hospital leaders to "help" Shulkin. In an article in USA Today, Shulkin said that he favors outsourcing some care to the private sector, which could also indicate trouble to come.[113]

Speaking at his Senate confirmation hearing on February 1, 2017, Shulkin said he opposed any VHA privatization. Many VHA observers worry that actions the administration has taken will present him with serious challenges. Although Trump did not appoint a supporter of the CVA as Secretary, Darin Selnick and other would be privatizers now hold top policy positions in the VHA's Office of Policy and Planning in Washington, D.C. Plus the VHA will face another threat in Congressional efforts to reintroduce bills, like those described earlier, that make the Choice program (which ends in August of 2017) permanent and eliminate restrictions on veteran use of non-VHA healthcare providers.

As undersecretary for health, Shulkin will also be saddled with a VA hiring freeze that will make his job much more difficult and has made the working environment at the VA extremely chaotic. When Trump announced his freeze on federal hiring on Monday, January 23, 2017, it did not exempt the VA. The VHA has over 41,000 unfilled positions throughout its system. Shulkin said that continued progress in providing high-quality care as well as in reducing wait times will depend on filling those positions.

To provide care, the VHA, like any other hospital system, must be able to expeditiously hire people when someone dies, retires, or leaves the system for employment elsewhere. (This is a big problem in the VHA, which for regulatory and budgetary reasons, does not offer salaries that are competitive with the private sector). Politicians have been urging the VHA to expeditiously fire any incompetent or employees guilty of wrong-doing. When they do, the positions left vacant must also be filled.

Under Trump's initial order, the VHA would not have been able to hire a single new primary-care physician, psychiatrist, nurse, nurse-practitioner, physical therapist, social worker, or counselor. It would not have been able to hire another urologist or cardiologist to help deal with the epidemic of Agent Orange–related prostate cancer or heart disease, from which so many Vietnam veterans suffer. It wouldn't have been able to add a single new neurologist or psychologist to deal with the twin afflictions of TBI and PTSD—signature problems for the veterans of our wars in Iraq and Afghanistan.

The VHA would not have been able to fully staff its two suicide crisis hotlines—one in rural Canandaigua, New York, and a newly opened facility in Atlanta, Georgia. At the time of this writing, crisis lines are currently short 171 employees, of whom only 26 would directly respond and follow up on calls from veterans in crisis. Three thousand psychology interns who were waiting to find out if they would be hired for internships in the VHA were also worried about the freeze. The VHA depends on these interns to care for patients.

Keeping veterans healthy is also the work of other VHA employees. Housekeepers and janitors make sure hospitals are free of the dangerous germs that cause hospital-acquired infections. Lab and radiation technicians play a vital role in the process of diagnosing medical conditions. VA police are specially trained to deescalate crisis situations so that mentally ill veterans don't harm themselves or others or commit what is known as suicide by cop. Hiring such staff and filling many more positions were initially prohibited under the freeze.

Because of more protests from VSOs as well as members of Congress from both parties, the administration relented and, on Thursday, January

27, acting VA Secretary Robert D. Snyder sent out a memorandum that exempted many frontline and support positions from the freeze, as well as health professional trainees like psychology interns.[114] Many VA leaders, caregivers, and veterans' groups breathed a sigh of relief.

While the memorandum exempting many categories of VA staff was another triumph of VSO organizing, it nonetheless left out many other employees who make it possible for the system to fill its tripartite mission. It takes administrators, as well as human relations staff—neither of them exempt from the hiring freeze—to hire sufficient numbers of, as well as supervise, frontline caregivers and medical support staff to meet the urgent healthcare needs of veterans. Under the Trump freeze, these positions, when they become vacant, will die. That will make VHA hiring delays even longer and the agency's already bureaucratic hiring process even more cumbersome.

The VHA also depends on researchers and research assistants to fulfill its mission to conduct cutting-edge research. The current freeze has generated considerable uncertainty over who can and cannot be hired to assist with this research.

In August 2016 the VHA opened the 61,000-square-foot Simulation, Learning, Education, and Research Network (SimLEARN), which uses high-technology simulations to enhance healthcare training and outcomes. Medical simulation is now recognized as critical to the delivery of high-quality, safe patient care. The taxpayers' $20-million investment has produced one of the ten largest medical simulation facilities in the country. But now, under the Trump freeze, SimLEARN cannot hire educational technicians, curriculum developers, simulation operators, researchers, or project managers.

Moreover, the VA's two Veterans Crisis Lines may now hire emergency responders but not other staff important to helping potentially suicidal veterans. Hiring staff to help the VHA fulfill the mandate of the Comprehensive Addiction and Recovery Act, as of this writing, is also frozen.[115] As one administrator told me, "We are in limbo and may have to renege on offers to candidates who have already been selected."

Another casualty of the VA hiring freeze: more delays for veterans trying to process claims at the chronically understaffed Veterans Benefits Administration. This agency determines whether a veteran has a service-connected disability and is therefore eligible for compensation and access to such VHA services as housing assistance, home loans, vocational rehabilitation, and educational benefits. Veterans have complained for years about delays at the Veterans Benefits Administration. These waits are about to get a lot longer.

Things will get even worse for veterans if Trump and congressional Republicans repeal the Affordable Care Act (ACA). Carrie Farmer, a health policy researcher at the RAND Corporation, pointed out that three million veterans enrolled in the VHA actually receive healthcare through employer-based plans or ACA exchanges. Farmer said she did not know how many of those veterans would flood into the VHA if the ACA were repealed. "I would expect that the number of veterans using VA healthcare will increase, which will only provide a further challenge for VA to provide timely and accessible care," she told NPR's Quil Lawrence in a radio interview.[116] With more vets seeking care, and not enough professionals to serve them, access will only get worse, and veterans' frustration will mount.

Faced with what will certainly be continued threats, veterans of all kinds must defend the thousands of VHA employees whose special expertise cannot be replicated through private-sector outsourcing without reducing the quality of care. I have observed these caregivers at work in more than twenty-five hospitals and clinics across the country. I have sat in on meetings with patients, therapy sessions, and home visits and seen VHA staff in action in rehabilitation and mental health facilities and many other settings. Nurses, physicians, social workers, psychologists, clerks, and many other VHA staff—including administrators—embody a commitment to serving patients often missing in other healthcare systems because of the way the latter are structured and run.

Even VHA staff members from civilian backgrounds see their professional practice as a calling, not just a career. As Rebecca Shunk, an internist at the San Francisco VA Health Care System, told me, "I didn't go to work at the VA to devote my life to veterans, but the minute I saw my first veteran patient, I knew this was my life's work." Many VHA staff, like Shunk, could earn more in private-sector jobs, yet they choose to remain at the side of those who served in uniform.

For Shunk and many others, one unanticipated and demoralizing reward for this life of service has been endlessly negative, factually inaccurate, and unfair media coverage. Intentionally or not, that VHA bashing in the press helped lay the groundwork for current political efforts to dismantle the VHA and steer veterans elsewhere. Amplified by the media, Donald Trump's own ignorant and insensitive remark about veterans with emotional problems has already damaged VHA efforts to destigmatize mental illness and encourage more vets to sign up for much-needed treatment.[117] On top of all this comes the chaos of the new hiring freeze, which means that, instead of spending time on patient care, administrators, researchers, and clinicians must try to figure out whether they will have the staff to deliver that care and beg for additional exemptions.

One chief of medical staff at a large VHA medical center observed privately that no other hospital system could be expected to conduct business in such a chaotic environment. This physician, who asked not to be named, worried that news of the freeze would also discourage people from even applying for jobs at the system. Given the choice between a job offer from the VHA and a private-sector employer, the physician wondered, who would choose to work in a place where the future is so uncertain?

All of this confusion will certainly impact services. But maybe that's the point. The worse things get at the VA, the more justification Trump will have to push for his real goal: privatization—despite the opposition of the vast majority of veterans and VSOs.

Fortunately, the ranks of the VHA are filled with people who are not "summer soldiers" or "sunshine patriots" in the field of healthcare delivery. Determined to continue providing "the best care anywhere," they have remained at their posts despite political attacks, media derision, understaffing, and the daily challenge of dealing with patients whose wounds, both mental and physical, are often difficult to heal. All who are concerned with veterans' health and the future of American healthcare must join with veterans' advocates to build on the nation's seventy-year investment in one of the great healthcare systems in the world. If the critical mission of their agency is undermined by Trump or Congress, Americans who have no connection to veterans will lose a shining model of coordinated, team-based, integrated care—a genuine community of care—that is largely unavailable in the private sector. But of course, the biggest losers of all will be the millions of veterans and their families who have sacrificed their health to serve a nation that too often seems unwilling to continue caring for them.[118]

APPENDIX A

From: [redacted]
To: Commission on Care
Subject: [EXTERNAL] Iraq War Veteran Date: Sunday, April 17, 2016
1:57:49 AM

Dear Commission on Care Members
I writing this in hopes to make you understand that the VA is more than a place that Veterans just get their health care at. Also I hope that my story will make you understand that the VA is more than worth saving because the VA saved ME! My name is and I am a Army OIF/OEF Veteran and have been getting my care at the Clement J Zablocki Va Medical Center in Milwaukee, WI since 2008. While I do understand that the VA has many issues and flaws but the issues are worth fixing by keeping Veteran health care within the VA system. First I want to start by saying that being a veteran is a brotherhood and going to the VA keeps us connected to each other. The VA is the only place that some of us feel safe and not out of place. The VA is the only place where I can always find someone that understands me and what I have gone through. Going to the VA is bigger than my health care but is is a place where I am never alone and hopefully my story will give you some understanding because it was the VA that made sure I knew that.

My VA story begins with me coming home from Iraq in 2007. After coming home from Iraq I was s member of Army Reserve and on a drill weekend we were told to report the drill hall because there was staff from the VA Medical Center that wanted to reach out and sign up anyone that has just return for combat for VA benefits. When I went though my demobilization process I was ordered to do this when I got back home so I did. Because I already signed up for care I didn't think that I need to see them but they wanted to meet with me regardless. They were both mental health providers and wanted to ask about my transition home. I began to rant and rage telling them that I thought I was going crazy. I knew something was wrong but I didn't know what. I knew something in me changed and I felt like a stranger to myself. I couldn't sleep at night, I was hearing gun fire in my sleep, waking up looking for my rifle, getting up and putting on my uniform during thunder storms. I was angry all the time with inappropriate outburst, having crying spells. My brain was always going and I couldn't figure out how to shake this out of my head. Because I didn't understand myself and didn't know who I was anymore, I started to drink to try to cope with this person I have become. One of the providers was a nurse that has served in a combat hospital in Afghanistan and could that I was in pain. He told me that he would have someone follow up with me to get started in my care and sit down with me to set up what I need. But all I thought was that I needed to just suck it up and drive on.

One day I received a call from an amazing social worker informing me that I was assigned to him and that he wanted to set up an appointment to get me started in my VA care. So I set up the appointment with him knowing that I didn't want to come in. I didn't want to come in because I was on a path of killing myself and I didn't see the need for VA care. On the day of the appointment I was mark as a no show because I was drunk and in my basement. The next day I received another phone call from the social worker informing me that I missed my appointment. He informed me of the importance of making my appointments and that I needed to come in. So we set up another appointment and I did the same thing and no showed again. Again my social worker called me and said the some thing "I need to make my appointments and so forth". I did this process for about over a month with me no showing and him calling. Finally I had enough and said okay I will come in if you stop calling me. So I made the appointment but this time I showed up because that weekend I found myself drunk in my basement with a rope around my neck ready to kill myself. Standing in my basement not knowing what is happening to me "I told myself why don't I go to this appointment and see what happens before I end it". And that was the start of the VA Health Care Saving my life. Not just mine but many Veterans like me that I met on my journey at the VA of figuring out who I was and what happened to the person I used to be.

Now you know a part of my journey with the VA Medical Center. I want to ask this committee since we know whats wrong with the VA do you know what is right? What is write is that my experience is something that comes with much sacrifice and the VA is the only place I feel safe with it. I am surrounded by men and women that know what serving our country really means. the VA is the place that I am surrounded by men and women that really understand the cost to keep this country safe. I like to remind you it was a combat veteran provider that saw my pain because he knew where I got it from and knew the journey to help me find some peace. With all due respect but this will be dishonoring the men and women that are willing to lay down theirs lives for this by taking away or closing locations that belongs to them. While I do agree that the Va needs reform but how about hiring VA executives that truly understand what it means when Abraham Lincoln said "To care for him who shall have borne the battle and for his widow, and his orphan". How about increasing the number of VA executives that are Veterans because they understand what being a veteran mean and what is takes to become one.

So to your solution of sending us to private healthcare providers is the wrong direction because the VA is filled with veteran and staff that have raised their right hands and said!

"I, do solemnly swear that I will support and defend the Constitution of the United States against all enemies, foreign and domestic; that I will bear true faith and allegiance to the same; and that I will obey the orders of the President of the United States and the orders of the officers appointed over me, according to regulations and the Uniform Code of Military Justice. So help me God."

There is no private health care provider office that can can offer me this type of care. So just fix our VA because it belongs to us not to the private sector.

Thank You Iraq Veteran

In mid-July 2016, I received this email.

Ms. Gordon,

My husband found out tonight that you posted the letter that he wrote to the Commission on VA Care. Let me start by stating that he had a very emotional reaction. At first it was confusion, then it was a lot of questions, and lastly it was relief.

His confusion came from finding the words he painstakingly wrote out for hours and hours on someone's website.

Questions came in many forms...how did she get access to my letter? Why would this person I don't know post my words on a public site? What is her stance on what the Commission is trying to accomplish? Did my words hurt or help the VA I cherish so much?

Relief came when he read other posts you had written to find out you agree with what he thinks and feels about VHA care.

There is no other Healthcare system that has the understanding or systems to treat the whole Veteran the way that the VA can. Each provider that my husband sees has access to charting from every other provider that sees him. From his Mental Health provider, his Dentist, his Primary Care provider, his Physical Therapy to the Opthamologist...they are all on the same page with his healthcare. Where else would he receive this type of treatment?

Where else would my husband be able to go and sit in a waiting room at a medical clinic and be comfortable knowing that the person sitting next to him, is just like him? 90 years old or 35 years old, they get each other. They are Veterans. They are one in the same. You speak to them and they all sound the same. They use the same words to describe their thoughts and feelings. They get it, they understand each other and what they have been through.

Where else are there providers who see Veterans all day long? They hear the same words day in and day out. They see the same look on their patient's faces. They deal with the same problems, patient after patient. Some of them are Veterans themselves. The VA providers get it too.

A couple of years ago, I sat with my husband in his Social Worker's office. We were signing papers for his Advance Directive and Power of Attorney for Healthcare. It was an emotional thing to do. The situation brought up a conversation with his Social Worker that I will never forget.

My husband thanked him that day. You see, this was the Social Worker that my husband wrote about in the email he sent to the Commission on VA Care. This man saved my husband's life. Had it not been for the persistent phone calls and letters that he sent to my husband...we would not have been sitting their signing papers that day. My husband would have taken his own life.

The three of us sat there that day in tears. My husband's tears were of gratitude to this man that didn't give up on him. My tears were for the same reason as well as the thought of possibly never having the opportunity to meet this amazing Veteran I am now honored to call my husband. His Social Worker's tears were from realizing the impact he has on the patients he is privileged to treat.

When I reflect on that day, and on what the Commission on VA Care is trying to accomplish, I think to myself...what about the other Veterans that would be thrown into a private healthcare system? A system where they will be just another number or statistic or dollar sign? They would never have the opportunity to receive the same care that my husband has had the privilege to receive.

I think about the 22 Veterans a day that commit suicide and I fear how that number could double or triple. The private sector does not have providers that would call again and again to make sure they make their appointments. They wouldn't waste their time on someone that is making them lose out the money when they no show to an appointment. They will fill those slots with patients that come and make their pockets heavier with money. The ones that keep their appointments. It would be a huge tragedy.

VHA treats the whole Veteran. They provide a clothing room that will put new clothes on a Veteran's back when he has been wearing the same clothes for weeks. They provide caseworkers that go out in below zero temperatures in the middle of the night to find the Veteran that is sleeping under a bridge and give him something to eat and a warm place for the night. They provide activities and outings for Veterans to teach them how to socialize again. They provide drug and alcohol treatment for the Veteran that has relapsed for the 5th time with the hope that this time it works. They provide medical care that is proven to be above and beyond the care that the private sector provides. But most of all, they provide the only place where the Veterans have found, since leaving the military, where they feel they belong.

My husband, my father, and any other Veteran I come in contact with all say the same thing about the VA. They love the care and treatment they receive, and it would be detrimental to them if they had to go elsewhere.

Thank you for being their voice. Thank you for standing up and listening to their words. Thank you for looking further into the things the media and the Commission are stating and for proving them wrong. Thank you for bringing a different light to the real truth behind the phenomenal care VHA provides to our nation's heroes.

You are to be commended for the time and commitment you are giving to this cause.

Sincerely,

A Veteran's Wife

Immediately after getting her email, I responded as follows.

Dear —,

I can't tell you how moved I am by your letter. I am a wordsmith, but words fail me in this instance. I am so glad you reached out and wrote to me. Let me explain why. But before I do, let me explain how I got your husband's letter and why I posted it on my blog.

When your husband submitted his letter to the Commission on Care, it became part of the public record. His name was redacted from it, but it was nonetheless made available to those of us covering the ongoing commission proceedings. It was such an important letter, as a public document explaining the importance of the veterans healthcare system, that I wanted it to reach a wider audience rather than be buried in proceedings where few would ever see it. So many veterans support the VHA. Their stories, insights, and concerns are buried in polling data and maybe in letters they send to politicians that we never see. The letter so eloquently stated the reality about the services provided by the VHA (facts that have been deliberately left out of the media attack on the system) that I felt it had to reach more people. I believe it should reach even more people than may have read it on my blog. I am so glad that, after your initial shock and dismay, you understand why I posted it and feel that its publication was important.

Let me now tell you why I am writing my book about VA healthcare. I am not a veteran; no one in my family has ever been a veteran. Some of my friends are vets, but not many. I began writing about VHA healthcare because I think it is often the best in America. I have spent thirty years writing about the broken American healthcare system. I know what kind of care most of us get—if we are lucky enough to have any health insurance at all. I have had the good fortune to have excellent health insurance—the best. But it is fragmented and unaccountable, with doctors and nurses who want to do the right thing but aren't given the time or resources to do it. So when I began learning more about the VHA, I wanted to write about the great models of care it provides. I started going to different VHAs and observing care there. And I was so impressed. Physicians and nurses, mental health professionals, clerks, all actually talk to each other. Moreover, they are given time to talk to each other. In the ten-minute visit primary care providers are allotted in the private sector, this rarely happens, even if providers want it to. Where is the time to talk to the patient, take a history, make a diagnosis, teach the patient about meds and treatments, and talk to the patient's other caregivers? It doesn't exist. The patient or family member has to be the care coordinator and care integrator because private-sector providers don't know how to do it, don't have the mechanisms with which to communicate with one another—the electronic medical record you mention, for example—and aren't rewarded for doing it because they aren't on salary but do piecework, and there is no money in interdisciplinary communication.

Plus, did you know this? Preventable medical mistakes are the third leading cause of death in the United States. Nearly 400,000 people die a year who could be alive today, and another 1.5 million are injured. I have suffered mightily because of this. Obviously, I didn't die from a preventable medical error, but ten years ago, I had a very bad complication after surgery and am suffering with it to this day. There was no way to hold anyone accountable because no lawyer would take the case—it wasn't serious enough, even though it was pretty darn serious to me. There was no congressperson to turn to, no congressional hearing at which I could air my grievance in the hope that problems in that hospital would be remedied so another patient would not suffer as I did. My problem was invisible, and that doctor and hospital proceeded to make mistake after mistake, and patients continued to suffer without any risk of media or government scrutiny. As you have seen on my blog, I also write about patient safety and teamwork, and the only place I have seen real teamwork in action is at the VHA.

So I began writing my book because I wanted to show all Americans that the VHA is a model not only for veteran care but for healthcare in general. When I started writing my book about VHA care several years ago, I was unfamiliar with the very specific problems of veterans. Since immersing myself in the VHA, I have been deeply impressed (and again, words fail me here) by the breadth and depth of problems veterans have—most of which are either acquired or exacerbated by exposures and experiences related to their military service. These problems are so many and so complex that, I now understand, they can only be dealt with by staff with extensive understanding and expertise in military culture and health.

Many of the best intentioned private-sector providers want to "do their bit" to help veterans without really understanding that you can't just pitch in an hour or two or have good intentions; you need special expertise to deal with—indeed, even to recognize—the problems veterans have. This is why the VHA is so important. Of course, the VHA has problems, most of which have to do with underfunding, micromanagement at the top, and the toxic environment Congress and the media have created. Congress has also given the VHA very limited resources to tell veterans and the public about the good things it does and the innovations it pioneers every day. The VHA is also prohibited from marketing. So you may read a billboard or see ads telling you how great the Cleveland Clinic is, but you will never learn about the San Francisco or Milwaukee or Boston VHA.

This is why more people need to hear from people like you and your husband. Many polls about VHA care register the fact that veterans value its services. Numbers don't move people to action, don't change the media narrative, and don't invade the heart and soul. Stories do.

Those attacking the VHA use the story of the veteran who doesn't like the VHA—and, as with any healthcare system, there are sometimes good reasons to complain. Sadly, these complaints are promoted without analysis or nuance. The larger questions are rarely asked: If there are problems in the VHA, why do they exist, and how does the VHA compare to private-sector healthcare (assumed, in this narrative, to be flawless and the very best in every way)?

Again, I want to thank you for your letter. Even if we never speak—and I certainly hope we will—it has meant more to me than you can imagine.

ACKNOWLEDGMENTS

So many people have helped me with this book that it is impossible to acknowledge all of them. I want to say a blanket thank you to all the veterans, VA staff, and many others who helped me learn about the healthcare system and understand veterans' issues and health conditions.

I want to give special thanks to the following people.

This book would not have been possible without the initial encouragement and support of Senator Bernie Sanders and Rajiv Jain, then assistant deputy undersecretary for patient care services at the VHA. Rebecca Shunk at the VA Health Care System in San Francisco also inspired me to undertake this project. William Outlaw and the compassionate and devoted Maureen McCarthy paved the way for me to observe caregivers all over the system. I also want to thank the many public affairs officers who spent so many hours organizing my visits. These include Judi Cheary, Matthew Coulson, Pamela Redmond, Pallas Wahl, Cynthia Butler, David Martinez, Naaman Horn, Michael Hill Thomas, Tara Ricks, Paul Coupaud, Penny Craft, and many others. Plus I want to thank then Undersecretary for Health David Shulkin for removing obstacles along the way.

I want to give special thanks to my editors, Robert Kuttner and Eliza Newlin Carney, at The American Prospect. As soon as I talked with them almost two years ago, they recognized the importance of doing systematic coverage of the VHA and assigned me to the VHA as my beat. They have continued to support my work. The team I have worked with at The Prospect—Amanda Teuscher, Gabrielle Gurley, and Sam Ross-Brown—have helped strengthen my work, as all good editors do.

I also want to thank Randy Shaw and Beyond Chron for publishing my many pieces. Randy was such a champion. Phillip Longman and Paul Glastris at The Washington Monthly also continually supported my work. Thank you especially to Phil for all the time you put into clarifying so many complex issues. Thanks also go to Michael Blecker and Bradford Adams and the staff at Swords to Plowshares. Peter Dickinson, Joy Ilem, and Garry Augustine at Disabled American Veterans have been invaluable, as has Rick Weidman at Vietnam Veterans of America. Thank you also to Sherman Gillums Jr. of Paralyzed Veterans of America and Bill Rausch of Got Your Six. I want to thank Beto O'Rourke and Mark Takano for constantly standing up for veterans on the House Veterans' Affairs Committee and tweeting my articles.

When he was at Bernie Sanders' office working on veterans' affairs, Steve Robertson was indefatigable in answering my many questions about the byzantine eligibility requirements and many other issues that impact the system.

I am also grateful to Marilyn Park, Brett Copeland, and Ian Hoffmann at AFGE for their work on these issues and their clarifications along the way. My old friend Hans Von Blankensee walked me through the history of the VA's world-class health information technology system, and Ross Koppel shed light on contemporary HIT issues.

The devoted staff I have met at VA facilities all over the country have served veterans by helping me understand their problems and concerns. My cousin Andrew Budson housed me and drove me through literal blizzards to observe care at the VHA in Boston. Cecelia McVey helped organize a visit to a special program training physicians and nurses to work together. Erin Finley in San Antonio explained the role anthropology plays in the system. I cannot give enough thanks to Harold Kudler for taking time to explain the role of mental health in the system. Thanks also go to Matt Friedman, Paula Schnurr, Terry Keane, and Andrew Pomerantz. Thomas Kirchberg in Memphis has talked me through a host of issues, and Edgardo Padin-Rivera in Cleveland illuminated the readjustment problems combat veterans like himself experience. Thomas Horvath provided insights into high-level VA administration. My dear friend Kate McPhaul gave me not only bed and breakfast but information on the work the VA does protecting workers on the job. I also want to thank Jeff Kixmiller, Liza Katz, and Sasha Best at the Martinez CBOC and Rebecca Stallworth in Sacramento and Cathy Coppolillo in Milwaukee.

My special thanks go to the many people at the San Francisco VA Health Care System, where I spent so much time. The system's director, Bonnie Graham, has worked with her leadership team to create one of the best medical centers in the country. Russell Lemle has been critical to the success of this project, as was John McQuaid. Thank you also to Keith Armstrong, Thomas Neylan, Karen Parko, Shira Maguen, Karen Seal, Susannah Fryer, Ian Ramsey, Jennifer Manuel, Brian Borsari, and Ben Emmert-Aronson and Joan Zweben. The palliative care and geriatric team—Eric Widera, Patrice Villars, Barb Drye, Caroline Talmadge, Erin

Bowman, and Anne Kelly—as well as Michael Harper, Heather Nye, Kathryn Eubanks, and Jessica Eng gave me insights into the intricate web of care at the VHA. I also want to thank the many staff in primary care, like Terry Keene and Anna Strewler, among others, who allowed me to observe their practice. Thanks particularly to Maya Dulay, Allison Ludwig, James Caldwell, Charles Filanosky, and Carolyn Wong. I also want to thank Rebecca Brienza, as well as Laurie Harkness and the staff at the Errera Center. Thank you to Charlene Phipps, Christina Kim, and Heather Freitag and staff in the Home Based Primary Care program in San Francisco. Thank you also to Bill Collins in Oakland.

Many veterans helped me along the way. My dear friend Louis Kern has been with me from day one. I also want to thank Ruth Johnson and Frank Hamilton, as well as Joshua Wilder Oakley.

Matt Rothschild helped me shape a series of disparate articles into what I hope is a coherent whole, and Denise Logsdon polished the manuscript. I also want to thank David Cole for his support and Lisa Hill for quick cover turnaround.

Fran Benson, Martyn Beeny, and Dean Smith at Cornell University Press deserve special thanks for bending deadlines to make this book possible. I cannot thank them enough. And I am deeply moved that Ken Kizer took the time to write such a powerful foreword.

In an amazing coincidence, my daughter Jessica Early worked as a nurse-practitioner at the VA Medical Center in West Haven, Connecticut. Wise beyond her years, she helped me grasp the many nuances of what it means to give care to veterans with complex health issues. My daughter Alex Early was, as ever, a huge cheerleader. And then, of course, there is my husband, Steve Early, who is himself a veteran of sorts—of living with me and my relentless requests for his editorial advice. He has made me a better writer—not to mention a better person—for too many decades to count.

NOTES

1. Kenneth W. Kizer and Ashish K. Jha. "Restoring Trust in VA Health Care." NEJM 371 (2014): 295–297. http://www.nejm.org/doi/full/10.1056/NE-JMp1406852

2. Phillip Longman. *The Best Care Anywhere: Why VA Health Care Would Work Better for Everyone.* Berrett-Koehler Publishers, 2012.

3. American College of Physicians. "The Role of the Department of Veterans Affairs in Geriatric Care." Position Paper, *Annals of Internal Medicine* 15, no. 11 (1991): 896–900. https://www.acponline.org/acp_policy/policies/role_of_veterans_affairs_department_in_geriatric_care_1999.pdf

4. Veterans Administration. "VA Campus Toolkit: What Is the VITAL Initiative?" http://www.mentalhealth.va.gov/studentveteran/vital.asp#sthash.mzOULaKW.dpbs

5. Austin Fract. "You Mean I Don't Have to Show Up. The Promise of Telemedicine." *The New York Times.* May 16, 2016. https://www.nytimes.com/2016/05/17/upshot/you-mean-i-dont-have-to-show-up-the-promise-of-telemedicine.html

6. Jon Hamilton. "Pentagon Shelves Blast Gauges Meant to Detect Battlefield Brain Injuries." *NPR Morning Edition,* December 20, 2016. http://www.npr.org/sections/health-shots/2016/12/20/506146595/pentagon-shelves-blast-gauges-meant-to-detect-battlefield-brain-injuries

7. Swords to Plowshares. "Underserved: How the VA Wrongfully Excludes Veterans with Bad Papers." National Veterans Legal Services Program. Veterans Legal Clinic, Legal Services Center of Harvard Law School. March 2016.

8. Congressional Budget Office. CBO Comparing the Costs of the Veterans' Health Care System with Private-Sector Costs, December 2014, 5. https://www.cbo.gov/sites/default/files/113th-congress-2013-2014/reports/49763-VA_Healthcare_Costs.pdf

9. The Cleveland Clinic Foundation. Department of the Treasury. Internal Revenue Service. Form 990. 2014, 7. https://my.clevelandclinic.org/ccf/media/Files/About/financial-statements/form-990/2014/2014-form-990.pdf?la=en

10. Andrea K. Walker. "Hopkins workers set to strike Friday after impasse on negotiations." *Baltimore Sun,* June 24, 2014. http://www.baltimoresun.com/health/bs-hs-hopkins-contract-stalemate-

20140624-story.html

11. This chapter was taken from the following articles: "Unfriendly Fire: Despite ideological attacks and underfunding, the Veterans Health Administration is a model public system." Tapped: The Prospect Group Blog, October 30, 2015. http://prospect.org/article/why-veterans-health-system-better-you-think

12. U.S. Department of Veterans Affairs. "The Origin of the VA Motto." http://www.va.gov/opa/publications/celebrate/vamotto.pdf Accessed January 1, 2015.

13. Assessment B (Health Care Capabilities). RAND Corporation, September 1, 2015. http://www.va.gov/opa/choiceact/documents/assessments/assessment_b_health_care_capabilities.pdf

14. V. Nuti Sudhakar et al. "Association of Admission to Veterans Affairs Hospitals vs Non–Veterans Affairs Hospitals with Mortality and Readmission Rates among Older Men Hospitalized with Acute Myocardial Infarction, Heart Failure, or Pneumonia." *JAMA* 315, no. 6 (2016):582–592. http://jamanetwork.com/journals/jama/fullarticle/2488309

15. Elizabeth Yano and Lori Bastian. Women's Veteran Research, VA Women's Health Research Network, 2011. http://www.va.gov/womenvet/docs/2011summit/WomenVeteransResearch.pdf

16. Veterans Health Administration. Veterans Affairs, American Customer Satisfaction Index. Customer Satisfaction Outpatient Survey, 2013. http://www.va.gov/health/docs/VA2013OutpatientACSI.pdf. Veterans Health Administration. Veterans Affairs, American Customer Satisfaction Index, Customer Satisfaction Inpatient Survey, 2013. http://www.va.gov/health/docs/VA2013InpatientACSI.pdf

17. Joe Carlson. "Cleveland Clinic cases highlight flaws in safety oversight." *Modern Health Care,* June 7, 2014. http://www.modernhealthcare.com/article/20140607/MAGAZINE/306079939

18. Brandon Glenn. "Cleveland Clinic's Millionaire's Club Adds 2 in 2010, grows to 15 members." *MedCity News*, December 22, 2011. http://medcitynews.com/2011/12/cleveland-clinic-millionaires-club-adds-2-in-2010-grows-to-15-members/ Accessed December 15, 2016. Cleveland Clinic, IRS, 7.

19. Alicia Mundy. "The VA Isn't Broken—Yet." Washington Monthly, March, April, May 2016. http://washingtonmonthly.com/magazine/marapr-may-2016/the-va-isnt-broken-yet/

20. Bridge Project. http://bridgeproject.com/app/uploads/Concerned-Veterans-for-America-Report.pdf

21. This chapter contains material originally published in "Privatization Won't Fix the VA," *Boston Globe,* May 27, 2014. https://www.bostonglobe. com/opinion/2014/05/27/privatization-won-fix/OyQgHoer1VXFNfkQ-Tyo1tI/story.html "VA Outperforms Private Sector on Key Measures." Report, *American Prospect,* November 20, 2015. http://prospect.org/article/report-va-outperforms-private-sector-key-measures "Why Privatizing the VA health care system is a bad idea." *Boston Globe Sunday Magazine,* February 17, 2016. https://www.bostonglobe.com/magazine/2016/02/17/ why-privatizing-health-care-system-bad-idea/2PyB5Dz36pdahjwVFr3p3M/ story.html "The future of the Veterans Health Administration." *BMJ*, April 29, 2016. http://blogs.bmj.com/bmj/2016/04/29/suzanne-gordon-the-future-of-the-veterans-health-administration/

22. Richard A. Oppel, Jr. "V.A. Official Acknowledges Link between Delays and Patient Deaths." *New York Times*, September 17, 2014. https://www. nytimes.com/2014/09/18/us/va-officials-acknowledge-link-between-delays-and-patient-deaths.html?_r=0

23. Dave Phillips. "In Unit Stalked by Suicide, Veterans Try to Save One Another." *New York Times*, September 19, 2015. http://www.nytimes. com/2015/09/20/us/marine-battalion-veterans-scarred-by-suicides-turn-to-one-another-for-help.html

24. Janet E. Kemp. "Suicide Rates in VHA Patients through 2011 with Comparisons with Other Americans and Other Veterans through 2010." Veterans Health Administration, January 2014. http://www.mentalhealth.va.gov/ docs/suicide_data_report_update_january_2014.pdf

25. Personal communication by email, August 15, 2016.

26. Pew Research Center, Politics & Policy. "Beyond Distrust: How Americans View Their Government." November 23, 2015. http://www.people-press.org/2015/11/23/beyond-distrust-how-americans-view-their-government/

27. Paul Ryan. Press release. "The VA's Problem Isn't Funding – It's Outright Failure. June 25, 2015. http://www.speaker.gov/press-release/boehner-va-s-problem-isn-t-funding-it-s-outright-failure

28. Jeff Miller. "Fix the VA, Mr. President." *Pittsburgh Post-Gazette*, July 21, 2015. https://veterans.house.gov/story-type/editorials/fix-va-mr-president

29. Independent Assessment. Assessment B Health Care Capabilities. RAND Corporation, September 1, 2015. http://www.va.gov/opa/choiceact/documents/assessments/assessment_b_health_care_capabilities.pdf

30. Peter S. Hussey et al. "Resources and Capabilities of the Department of Veterans Affairs to Provide Timely and Accessible Care to Veterans." RAND

Corporation, 2015. http://www.rand.org/pubs/research_reports/RR1165z2. htmlhttp://www.rand.org/pubs/research_reports/RR1165z2.html

31. U.S. Department of Veterans Affairs. "The Joint Commission releases results of surveys of the VA health care system." http://www.blogs.va.gov/ VAntage/29825/joint-commission-releases-results-surveys-va-health-care-system/

32. This story includes material from the following articles. "Report: VA Outperforms Private Sector on Key Measures," American Prospect, November 20, 2015. http://prospect.org/blog/tapped/studies-show-veter-ans-health-care-improving "Studies Show Veterans Health Care Improv-ing," Tapped: The Prospect Group Blog, August 16, 2016. http://prospect. org/article/report-va-outperforms-private-sector-key-measures

33. Steve Eder and Dave Phillips. "Faith in Agency Clouded Bernie Sanders' V.A. Response." *New York Times*, February 6, 2016. http://www.nytimes. com/2016/02/07/us/politics/faith-in-agency-clouded-bernie-sanderss-va-response.html

34. Wade Miller. "Sanders' Veteran Bill Asphyxiates the VA System." Her-itage Foundation for America, February 24, 2014. http://heritageaction. com/2014/02/sanders-veteran-bill-asphyxiates-va-system/

35. Stephen K. Trynosky. "Beyond the iron triangle: implications for the Vet-erans Health Administration in an uncertain policy environment." School of Advanced Military Studies, United States Army Command and General Staff College. Fort Leavenworth, Kansas, 2014-02. http://cgsc.contentdm. oclc.org/cdm/ref/collection/p4013coll3/id/3283

36. Arti Parikh-Patel et al. "Disparities in Stage at Diagnosis, Survival, and Quality of Cancer Care in California by Source of Health Insurance." UC Davis Institute for Population Health Improvement. https://www.ucdmc. ucdavis.edu/iphi/resources/1117737_CancerHI_100615.pdf

37. This article first appeared in Tapped: The Prospect Group Blog as "The Times Sloppy Reporting on Sanders and Veterans Health." February 8, 2016. http://prospect.org/blog/tapped/times%E2%80%99s-sloppy-report-ing-sanders-and-veterans-health

38. Terri Tanielian et al. "Ready to Serve: Community-Based Provider Capaci-ty to Deliver Culturally Competent, Quality Mental Health Care to Veterans and Their Families." RAND Corporation, 2014, 2. http://www.rand.org/ pubs/research_reports/RR806.html

39. Tanielian et al., "Ready to Serve," 11.

40. This article appeared in Tapped: The Prospect Group Blog as "McCain Pulls a Bait-and-Switch on Vets," June 9, 2016, http://prospect.org/blog/

tapped/mccain-pulls-bait-and-switch-vets

41. Drew Griffin. "VA Secretary Disneyland-wait time comparison draws ire." CNN, May 23, 2016. http://www.cnn.com/2016/05/23/politics/veterans-affairs-secretary-disneyland-wait-times/

42. Emilye Bell. "No Sec. McDonald, VA Wait Lists Don't Compare to Disney World." Concerned Veterans for America. May, 23, 2016. https://cv4a.org/sec-mcdonald-va-wait-lists-dont-compare-disneyworld/

43. Curt Mills. "VA Secretary Declines Apology for Disney Remark. U.S. News. May 24, 2016. http://www.usnews.com/news/articles/2016-05-24/mcdonald-stands-by-disney-remark

44. Tom LoBianco. "VA's McDonald apologizes for Disney waiting line comparison." CNN. May 24, 2016. http://www.cnn.com/2016/05/24/politics/bob-mcdonald-veterans-affairs-disney/

45. Fred Lee. "If Disney Ran Your Hospital: 9 1/2 Things You Would Do Differently." *Second River Healthcare*, 2004.

46. https://www.cms.gov/Medicare/Quality-Initiatives-Patient-Assessment-instruments/HospitalQualityInits/HospitalHCAHPS.html

47. Quint Studer. *The HCAHPS Handbook*. Firestarter Publishing, 2010.

48. Joe Carlson. "Cleveland Clinic cases highlight flaws in safety oversight." *Modern Health Care*, June 7, 2014. http://www.modernhealthcare.com/article/20140607/MAGAZINE/306079939

49. This was first published in Tapped: The Prospect Group Blog as "The Hidden Irony of GOP Outrage over the VA Secretary's Disney Comparison," May 31, 2016. http://prospect.org/blog/tapped/hidden-irony-gop-outrage-over-va-secretary%E2%80%99s-disney-comparison

50. Gail Collins. "Trump and Clinton Take Up Arms." *New York Times*, September 8, 2016. http://www.nytimes.com/2016/09/08/opinion/trump-and-clinton-take-up-arms.html?rref=collection%2Fcolumn%2Fgail-collins&action=click&contentCollection=opinion&region=stream&module=stream_unit&version=latest&contentPlacement=2&pgtype=collection&_r=0 Accessed December 31, 2016.

51. Gail Collins. "Trump and Clinton Take Up Arms." *New York Times*, September 8, 2016, published in *Seattle Times*. http://www.seattletimes.com/opinion/donald-trump-and-hillary-clinton-take-up-arms/ Accessed December 31, 2016.

52. Emily Wax-Thibodeaux. "VA spent $6.3 million on sculptures and fountains for their hospitals. Should they have?" *Washington Post,* October 9, 2015. https://www.washingtonpost.com/news/federal-eye/wp/2015/10/09/the-va-spent-6-3-million-on-sculptures-and-fountains-for-their-hospitals-

should-they-have/?utm_term=.d590578923b6

53. Naj Wikoff. "Cultures of Care: A Study of Arts Programs in U.S. Hospitals." Report for Americans for the Arts, November 2004. http://www.americansforthearts.org/sites/default/files/Arts%20and%20Healthcare%20Nov2004_0.pdf

54. Jennifer Finkel. "Contemporary art in medicine: the Cleveland Clinic art collection." *Cardiovascu Diagn Ther* 1, no. 1 (December 2011): 71–75. https://www.ncbi.nlm.nih.gov/pmc/articles/PMC3839134/

55. Laura Landro. "More Hospitals Use the Healing Powers of Public Art." *Wall Street Journal.* August 18, 2014. http://www.wsj.com/articles/more-hospitals-use-the-healing-powers-of-public-art-1408404629

56. Cleveland Clinic. Art Program. http://my.clevelandclinic.org/services/arts_medicine/art-program

57. Henry Ford Health System. Healing Arts. https://www.henryford.com/locations/west-bloomfield/visitors/healing-arts Accessed January 1, 2017.

58. This article appeared in *Washington Monthly blog,* "In Defense of Art in VA Hospitals," September 13, 2016. http://washingtonmonthly.com/2016/09/13/in-defense-of-art-in-va-hospitals/

59. Commission on Care. https://commissiononcare.sites.usa.gov/

60. Jeff Miller. Letter to Nancy Schlichting, March 14, 2016.https://www.scribd.com/doc/304881244/Letter-To-Chairwoman-Nancy-M-Schlichting#download

61. Mundy, "The VA Isn't Broken Yet."

62. Paul Glastris. "More on the VA 'Scandal' That Wasn't." Washington Monthly, March 17, 2016. http://washingtonmonthly.com/people/paul-glastris-2/

63. Suzanne Gordon notes of meeting.

64. This post appeared in Tapped: The Prospect Group Blog as House Veterans Affairs Chairman Blasts Health Care Commission Member. March 22, 2016. http://prospect.org/blog/tapped/house-veterans-affairs-chairman-blasts-health-care-commission-member

65. David Blom et al. "The Straw Man Document," March 18, 2016. https://commissiononcare.sites.usa.gov/files/2016/03/2016.3.18-Proposed-Strawman-Assessment-and-Recommendations.pdf

66. Association of VA Psychologist Leaders. Fact Sheet. "Comparison of VA to Community Health Care," Summary of Research 2000–2016. March 23, 2016. http://advocacy.avapl.org/pubs/FACT%20sheet%20literature%20review%20of%20VA%20vs%20Community%20Heath%20Care%2003%2023-16.pdf

67. Disabled American Veterans. "Setting the Record Straight." https://www.youtube.com/watch?v=VR2cbEYyugA

68. David J. Shulkin. "Beyond the VA Crisis—Becoming a High-Performance Network." *NEJM* 374 (2016):1003–1005. http://www.nejm.org/doi/full/10.1056/NEJMp1600307?af=R&rss=currentIssue&

69. This article appeared in Tapped: The Prospect Group Blog as "Group Drafts Secret Proposal to End Taxpayer-Funded Veteran Care," March 26, 2016. http://prospect.org/blog/tapped/group-drafts-secret-proposal-end-taxpayer-funded-veteran-care

70. Commission on Care. Final Report. June 30, 2016. https://commissiononcare.sites.usa.gov/files/2016/07/Commission-on-Care-_Final-Report_Cover.jpg

71. Darin S. Selnick and Stewart M. Hickey. Commission Report Dissent. June 30, 2016. http://www.stripes.com/polopoly_fs/1.417808.1467833835!/menu/standard/file/COC%20Commissioners%20Report%20Dissent%20063016122.pdf

72. Michael Blecker. Letter of Dissent. June 29, 2016. https://www.swords-to-plowshares.org/sites/default/files/Dissent%20Letter%20from%20Commissioner%20Michael%20Blecker%2006-29-2016.pdf Accessed June 30, 2016.

73. Cathy McMorris Rodgers. Website. "McMorris Rodgers Releases Draft VA Reform Legislation." June 7, 2016. https://mcmorris.house.gov/mcmorris-rodgers-releases-draft-va-reform-legislation/

74. Letter to Nancy Schlichting, Chair, VA Commission on Care. April 29, 2016. https://commissiononcare.sites.usa.gov/files/2016/05/Letter_from-VSOs-reChoice_2016-04-29.pdf Accessed May 1, 2016.

75. Association of VA Psychologist Leaders et al. Policy Brief re Commission on Care Final Report: Major Recommendation Ignores Data, Risks Veterans' Healthcare. July 22, 2016. http://advocacy.avapl.org/pubs/Health%20Care%20Professionals%20&%20Federal%20Unions%20Policy%20Brief%20July%202016%20Response%20to%20Commission%20on%20Care.pdf Accessed July 23, 2016.

76. Curt Devine and Drew Griffin. "Billions spent to fix VA didn't solve problems, made some issues worse." *CNN*, July 6, 2016. http://www.cnn.com/2016/07/05/politics/veterans-administration-va/ Accessed July 8, 2016.

77. "Heal the V.A. (But First, Do No Harm)." *New York Times*, July 7, 2016. http://www.nytimes.com/2016/07/07/opinion/heal-the-va-but-first-do-no-harm.html Accessed July 8, 2016.

78. Material in this chapter first appeared as "Report as Report: VHA Care Commission Recommends Private-Sector Options," *American Prospect,* July 12, 2016, http://prospect.org/article/report-vha-care-commission-rec-ommends-privatizing-some-services "Veterans' Groups: Don't Scrap the VA's Health Care System." Tapped: The Prospect Group Blog, May 6, 2016. http://prospect.org/blog/tapped/veterans%E2%80%99-groups-don%E2%80%99t-scrap-va%E2%80%99s-health-care-system

79. Blecker, Letter of Dissent.

80. Blecker, Letter of Dissent.

81. Kenneth W. Goodman et al. "Challenges in ethics, safety, best practices, and oversight regarding HIT vendors, their customers, and patients: a report of an AMIA special task force." *Journal of the American Medical Informatics Association* 18, no. 1. (2011): 77–81. http://jamia.oxfordjournals.org/content/18/1/77.short Accessed July 7, 2016.

82. Sean W. Smith and Ross Koppel. "Healthcare information technology's relativity problems: a typology of how patients' physical reality, clinicians' mental models, and healthcare information technology differ." Journal of the American Medical Informatics Association 21, no. 1 (2014): 117–131. http://jamia.oxfordjournals.org/content/21/1/117.short Accessed July 10, 2016.

83. Donna M. Zulman et al. "Evolutionary Pressures on the Electronic Health Record: Caring for Complexity." *JAMA* 316, no. 9 (2016): 923–924. http://jamanetwork.com/journals/jama/article-abstract/2545405 Accessed September 10, 2016.

84. Material for this chapter appeared in Tapped: The Prospect Group Blog as "Hill Hearing Spells Bad News for Veterans," September 12, 2016. http://prospect.org/blog/tapped/hill-hearing-spells-bad-news-veterans

85. This chapter was originally published in *Washington Monthly* as "A Conversation about the Commission on Care and the Future of the VA," July 14, 2016. http://washingtonmonthly.com/2016/07/14/a-conversation-about-the-commission-on-care-and-the-future-of-the-va/

86. This chapter appeared in Beyond Chron as "Will Trump Jeopardize VA Prostate Research?" January 3, 2016. http://www.beyondchron.org/will-trump-jeopardize-va-prostate-research/

87. 90198 *Federal Register* 81, no. 240 (Wednesday, December 14, 2016): Rules and Regulations.

88. Institute of Medicine. *The Future of Nursing: Leading Change, Advancing Health.* Washington, D.C.: National Academies Press. October 5, 2010.

89. AMA. "AMA statement on VA rule on advanced practice nurses." Decem-

ber 13, 2016. https://www.ama-assn.org/ama-statement-va-rule-advanced-practice-nurses

90. Suzanne Gordon and Edwin Herzog, producers. "How to Huddle." HIIP Productions, 2015. http://suzannecgordon.com/how-to-huddle/

91. Daniel Zwerdling. "At VA Hospitals, Training And Technology Reduce Nurses' Injuries." *NPR*, February 25, 2015, 4:33 PM ET. http://www.npr.org/2015/02/25/387298633/at-va-hospitals-training-and-technology-reduce-nurses-injuries

92. Material from this chapter appeared in Tapped: The Prospect Group Blog as "VHA Support for Nurse Practitioners Draws Fire from Medical Leaders," December 20, 2016. http://prospect.org/blog/tapped/vha-support-nurse-practitioners-draws-fire-medical-leaders

93. This article appeared in Beyond Chron as "VHA Researches the Brain at War," October 22, 2015. http://www.beyondchron.org/vha-researches-the-brain-at-war/

94. NCIRE. "The Brain at War," 2015. https://www.ncire.org/TheBrainat-War/2015_highlights/ Accessed January 5, 2017.

95. Bridge Project and VoteVets.org. "The Vets Group that Fights against Veterans." http://www.aflcio.org/Blog/Other-News/Report-Koch-Funded-Concerned-Veterans-for-America-Wants-to-Dismantle-VA-Cut-Veterans-Benefits

96. Chelsea C. Cook. "Veteran's suicide note goes viral; family demands better for veterans." CNN, July 6, 2013. http://www.cnn.com/2013/07/06/us/soldier-suicide-note/

97. Janet E. Kemp. "Suicide Rates in VHA Patients through 2011 with Comparisons with Other Americans and Other Veterans through 2010." Veterans Health Administration, January 2014. http://www.mentalhealth.va.gov/docs/suicide_data_report_update_january_2014.pdf

98. Tanielian et al, "Ready to Serve."

99. Katherine E. Watkins et al. "The Quality of Medication Treatment for Mental Disorders in the Department of Veterans Affairs and in Private-Sector Plans. *Psychiatric Services* 67, no. 4 (April 1, 2016): 391–396. http://ps.psychiatryonline.org/doi/10.1176/appi.ps.201400537

100. This article appeared in Beyond Chron as "The Problem of Gun-Related Suicides," March 8, 2016. http://www.beyondchron.org/the-problem-of-gun-related-suicides/

101. Leo Shane III. "Trump's comments on veterans mental health care spark new outrage." *Military Times,* October 3, 2016. http://www.militarytimes.com/articles/trump-comments-mental-health-controversy Accessed November 5, 2016.

102. David A. Fahrenthold. "Four months after fundraiser, Trump says he gave $1 million to veterans group." *Washington Post*, May 24, 2016. https://www.washingtonpost.com/news/post-politics/wp/2016/05/24/four-months-later-donald-trump-says-he-gave-1-million-to-veterans-group/?utm_term=.c01b29e15726 Accessed May 25, 2016.

103. Michael D. Shear. "Trump Weighs Letting Veterans Opt Out of V.A. Medical Care." *New York Times*, December 28, 2016. http://www.nytimes.com/2016/12/28/us/politics/trump-weighs-letting-veterans-opt-out-of-va-medical-care.html

104. Joe Davidson. "Gingrich urges Trump to take aim at the federal bureaucracy, starting with VA." *Washington Post*. December 16, 2016. https://www.washingtonpost.com/news/powerpost/wp/2016/12/16/gingrich-urges-trump-to-take-aim-at-the-federal-bureaucracy-starting-with-the-va/?utm_term=.c897e95b7028 Accessed December 16, 2016.

105. Arvik Roy. "Veterans Should Enjoy the Same Health Care Options as All Americans." *New York Times*, June 28, 2016. http://www.nytimes.com/roomfordebate/2016/06/28/should-the-veterans-health-care-system-be-privatized

106. Michelle Ye Hee Lee. "Democrats' misleading claim that Concerned Veterans for America wants to 'privatize' VA." *Washington Post,* December 7, 2016. https://www.washingtonpost.com/news/fact-checker/wp/2016/12/07/democrats-misleading-claim-that-concerned-veterans-for-america-wants-to-privatize-the-va/?utm_term=.ce58ef76ad9c Accessed December 10, 2016.

107. Paul Starr. "The Meaning of Privatization." *Yale Law and Policy Review* 6 (1988): 6–41. https://www.princeton.edu/%7Estarr/articles/articles80-89/Starr-MeaningPrivatization-88.htm Accessed December 9, 2016.

108. House Committee on Veterans Affairs. Press Release. "Miller Bill Would Enable Real Accountability for All VA Employees, Reform Appeals Process." July 6, 2016. https://veterans.house.gov/news/press-releases/miller-bill-would-enable-real-accountability-all-va-employees-reform-appeals Accessed January 17, 2017.

109. Harvey Feigenbaum, Jeffrey Henig, and Chris Hamnett. *Shrinking the State*. Cambridge: Cambridge University Press, 1998, 8.

110. David J. Shulkin. "Beyond the VA Crisis. Becoming a High-Performance Network." *NEJM* 374 (2016):1003–1005. http://www.nejm.org/doi/full/10.1056/NEJMp1600307#t=article Accessed January 10, 2017.

111. David J. Shulkin. "VA is Saving Veterans' Lives Every Day." *Omaha World-Herald*, October 11, 2016. http://www.omaha.com/opinion/david-j-

shulkin-va-is-saving-veterans-lives-every-day/article_748e0471-580b-5be3-800b-e47fc8816c64.html Accessed January 10, 2017.

112. David J. Shulkin. "Why VA Health Care Is Different." *Federal Practitioner* 33, no. 5 (2016): 9–11. http://www.mdedge.com/fedprac/article/108568/why-va-health-care-different

113. Donovan Slack. "Trump picks David Shulkin for secretary of Veterans Affairs." *USA Today*, January 11, 2017. http://www.usatoday.com/story/news/politics/2017/01/11/david-shulkin-trump-va-secretary/96444280/ Accessed January 16, 2017.

114. Department of Veterans Affairs. Memorandum. Exemption to Hiring Freeze under Presidential Memorandum dated January 23, 2017. January 27, 2017.

https://www.va.gov/opa/publications/factsheets/Signed-Exemption-to-Hiring-Freeze-Memo-with-Exempted-Occupations-1-27-2017.pdf

115. Comprehensive Addiction and Recovery Act. http://www.cadca.org/comprehensive-addiction-and-recovery-act-cara

116. Quil Lawrence. "Hiring Freeze and Obamacare Repeal Could Clobber Veterans Affairs." January 25, 2017. http://wamc.org/post/hiring-freeze-and-obamacare-repeal-could-clobber-veterans-affairs

117. Make The Connection. http://maketheconnection.net/what-is-mtc accessed January 10, 2017. American Psychological Association. "Veterans' Mental Health Care Emphasizes Recovery and Return to Full and Meaningful Lives." November 10, 2011. http://www.apa.org/news/press/releases/2011/11/recovery-return.aspx Accessed December 4, 2014.

118. Material in this chapter came from Tapped: The Prospect Group Blog as "Fact-Checking Fact-Checkers on Privatizing Vets' Health Care," and "For Once—Trump Makes the Right Cabinet Pick," January 13, 2017. "Hiring Freeze Spares Some at VA, But Shortages Still Loom." January 31, 2017. http://prospect.org/blog/tapped/fact-checking-fact-checkers-privatizing-vets%E2%80%99-health-care http://prospect.org/article/once-trump-makes-right-cabinet-pick http://prospect.org/article/hiring-freeze-spares-some-va-shortages-still-loom

SUZANNE GORDON

ABOUT THE AUTHOR

Suzanne Gordon is an award-winning journalist and author who writes about healthcare. She is the co-editor of the Culture and Politics of Health Care Work series at Cornell University Press and lectures all over the world about healthcare, patient safety, nursing, and teamwork. Her eighteen books include, *First, Do Less Harm: Confronting the Inconvenient Problems of Patient Safety, Beyond the Checklist: What Else Health Care Can Learn from Aviation Teamwork and Safety,* and *From Silence to Voice: What Nurses Know and Must Communicate to the Public.* She has spent the last three years observing and writing about veterans' healthcare and is writing a second book about clinical innovation and care at the Veterans Health Administration. in 2017, she was given the DAV's Special Recognition Award for her writing on veterans' health issues.

To read more about Suzanne please see her website and blog at suzannegordon.com

Look for Suzanne's next book on the Veterans' Health Administration in 2018, also from Cornell University Press.

Visit cornellpress.cornell.edu and use code 09sg17 to receive 30% off your next Suzanne Gordon book.

CPSIA information can be obtained
at www.ICGtesting.com
Printed in the USA
LVOW11s0044280418
575140LV00002BA/216/P